"Dr. Bailey's and Dr. Burch's decades-long contributions to the field of applied behavior analysis continue with this informative and empowering book for future Registered Behavior Technicians™. A heart-touching dedication page sets the tone and is a direct reflection of the energy and character of its authors. A must-read road map for those entering the field."

—**Erik Lovaas**, president of The Lovaas Center and Fundación Erik Lovaas Para el Autismo

"Once again, Bailey and Burch have provided the field with a timely and much-needed book. *The RBT® Ethics Code* will be of great benefit to Registered Behavior Technicians™ and those who supervise them. I see it as being an integral part of any training and supervisory effort and another layer of protection for the children and families served by entry-level behavior analytic practitioners."

—**Richard M. Foxx**, PhD, BCBA-D, Emeritus Professor of Psychology, Penn State University

"I'm delighted that Dr. Bailey and Dr. Burch have worked diligently to develop this book that is appropriate for use during the 40-hour training but also as a reference text for RBTs™ to utilize during their career. I believe it will be a great resource for our field and greatly appreciate the dedication to quality, ethical service that both authors have provided the field of behavior analysis."

—**Melissa L. Olive**, PhD, BCBA-D, LBA, Executive Director, Applied Behavioral Strategies

"Another winner from Bailey and Burch! *The RBT® Ethics Code* explains each of the 31 principles in easy-to-understand language, illustrated by actual ethical dilemmas drawn from Dr. Bailey's experience on ABAEthicsHotline.com, including suggested ways for RBTs™ to respond. A must read, not only for RBT® preparation, but also for employers and supervisors of RBTs™!"

—**Sharon Older**, PhD, BCBA-D, Executive Director, Adapt Behavioral Services, Florida

"Given the unparalleled growth in Registered Behavior Technicians™ (RBTs™), this Ethics Code book is a vital resource. Bailey and Burch logically tackle the ethics codes and provide detailed, clear, and practical scenarios throughout to assist RBTs™ in their work. It's a *'need to have'* book for RBTs™ and supervisors alike, and I'm excited to use it in my classes."

—**Kimberly A. Crosland**, PhD, BCBA-D,
Associate Professor, University
of South Florida

The RBT® Ethics Code

This practical textbook will enable students training to become Registered Behavior Technicians (RBTs™) to fully understand and follow the new RBT® Ethics Code administered by the Behavior Analyst Certification Board (BACB®).

Starting with an overview of the role of ethics and core ethical principles, subsequent chapters provide concrete guidance for each of the three sections of the RBT® Ethics Code: responsible conduct, responsibility to clients, and competence and service delivery. The authors then show correct and incorrect applications of each code item and provide practical examples and solutions for applying each section to everyday practice. Also included are test questions where RBTs™ can test themselves on their newfound knowledge, along with a glossary, the complete RBT® Code of Ethics, and suggested readings. Last, Appendix D, "Considerations and Conversation Starters," will help RBT™ trainers quickly focus on specific code items and presenting scenarios for discussion and role-plays.

This book is intended to serve as a primary text for the training of RBTs™ as well as a reference and study guide for these RBTs™ and their trainers.

Jon S. Bailey, PhD, BCBA-D, Emeritus Professor of Psychology at Florida State University, teaches graduate courses for behavior analysts. Dr. Bailey was a founding director of the Behavior Analyst Certification Board® and is past president of the Florida Association for Behavior Analysis and a Fellow of the American Psychological Association and the Association for Behavior Analysis International.

Mary R. Burch, PhD, BCBA-D, is a Board Certified Behavior Analyst®. Dr. Burch has more than 25 years of experience in developmental disabilities. She has been a behavior specialist, Qualified Mental Retardation Professional (QMRP), unit director, and consulting behavior analyst in developmental disabilities, mental health, and preschool settings.

The RBT® Ethics Code

Mastering the BACB© Ethical Requirements for Registered Behavior Technicians™

Jon S. Bailey and Mary R. Burch

Routledge
Taylor & Francis Group
NEW YORK AND LONDON

First published 2021
by Routledge
52 Vanderbilt Avenue, New York, NY 10017

and by Routledge
2 Park Square, Milton Park, Abingdon, Oxon, OX14 4RN

Routledge is an imprint of the Taylor & Francis Group, an informa business

Library of Congress Cataloging-in-Publication Data
Names: Bailey, Jon S., author. | Burch, Mary R., author.
Title: The RBT ethics code : mastering the BACB ethical requirements for registered behavior technicians / Jon S. Bailey, Mary R. Burch.
Other titles: Registered behavior technicians ethics code
Description: New York, NY : Routledge, 2020. | Includes bibliographical references and index. |
Identifiers: LCCN 2020006765 (print) | LCCN 2020006766 (ebook) | ISBN 9780367342630 (hbk) | ISBN 9780367415099 (pbk) | ISBN 9780367415099 (ebk)
Subjects: MESH: Behavior Analyst Certification Board. | Applied Behavior Analysis—ethics | Allied Health Personnel—ethics | Specialty Boards—organization & administration | Codes of Ethics | Certification | United States
Classification: LCC R724 (print) | LCC R724 (ebook) | NLM WM 21 | DDC 174.2/9073—dc23
LC record available at https://lccn.loc.gov/2020006765
LC ebook record available at https://lccn.loc.gov/2020006766

ISBN: 978-0-367-34263-0 (hbk)
ISBN: 978-0-367-41509-9 (pbk)
ISBN: 978-0-367-81492-2 (ebk)

Typeset in Minion
by Apex CoVantage, LLC

This book is dedicated to all of the honest, ethical RBTs who are on the frontline of the behavior analysis service-delivery system. As the new face of behavior analysis, these hardworking Registered Behavior Technicians often deserve far more credit than they receive for bringing the science of behavior to bringing the science of behavior to clients. Through their daily work, RBTs change the lives of countless children and adults who simply want to be accepted in society and achieve independence and happiness. We are elated that Registered Behavior Technicians have joined our profession and hope that this code of ethics will guide and protect them.

Jon S. Bailey, PhD, BCBA-D
Mary R. Burch, PhD, BCBA-D

Contents

Preface

EVOLUTION OF THIS BOOK AND HOW TO USE IT

In 1998, when the Behavior Analyst Certification Board (BACB) was formed, the first author was asked to be on the Board of Directors by Dr. Jerry Shook, the first CEO of the BACB. Dr. Bailey began teaching ethics and professional issues as part of the curriculum for the new master's program at the Panama City campus of FSU in 1999. At that time, there was no text on ethics for our field, and before long, students began to ask, "So, why don't you write the book?" This frequent question prompted us to write the first ethics book in 2005 as well as the "Second Expanded Edition" in 2011, when the Guidelines for Responsible Conduct were revised.

In 2009, the first author created an ethics "Hotline" in conjunction with the Association for Behavior Analysis. The Hotline began attracting attention and became the source of much of the material that was to be presented in subsequent texts (with permission of the writers and edited to protect identities, of course). In 2016, a new *Professional and Ethical Compliance Code for Behavior Analysts* was issued by the BACB, and the *3rd Edition of Ethics for Behavior Analysts* was published.

The title *Registered Behavior Technician*™ came into existence in 2014 in response to the overwhelming need for front-line therapists to work with Board Certified Assistant Behavior Analysts™ (BCaBAs®) and Board Certified Behavior Analysts® (BCBAs®). These "techs," as they are often called, have their own Task List and their own RBT Ethics Code.[1] In ongoing interactions with many RBTs, over time, it became clear that most were not aware that they now had their own Code, and those who knew there was a Code were unable to cite any items that were relevant to their daily work in ABA (Applied Behavior Analysis). It was then that the authors realized that a book written in easy-to-understand language just for RBTs was needed, and the spark for this book was ignited.

HOW TO USE THIS BOOK

This book is intended to be used as a textbook in a 40-hour RBT prep course or as a stand-alone book for new RBTs or individuals who might be thinking about becoming RBTs. We also believe this book will be a valuable reference on a daily basis for those working to accumulate their required supervision hours. For each of the 31 code items, there is a dedicated chapter in which we present a short description—*Quick Take*—of the code item in understandable language that captures the essence and the intent of the code item. This is followed by a series of realistic *Challenges* that present situations in which RBTs are likely to find themselves. Next we have *More Details*, where we provide background on the code item and delve into complications that are often associated with the item. Finally, we have in each chapter a *Test Yourself* section where we present a series of multiple-choice and true/false questions for readers to test their knowledge of the code items. The answers to the questions are in Appendix A. A unique feature of the book is Appendix D, "Considerations and Conversation Starters for RBT

1 Code items were designated for RBTs in the 2016 BACB Code of Ethics, but they were somewhat obscure and not precisely tailored to the needs and responsibilities of front-line therapists.

Trainers." In this helpful table, code topics are presented along with examples of ways to start a conversation related to specific code items.

We hope that the *Bill of Rights for RBTs* in Chapter 3 will be a valuable tool to help protect RBTs from intimidation and exploitation as they work with clients and handle conflicts that will inevitably arise.

Jon S. Bailey
Mary R. Burch

Acknowledgments

The authors would like to acknowledge the extraordinary contributions of *Loren Eighmie* and *Lindsey Ives* in the preparation and proofing drafts of this work. As practicing RBTs, Loren and Lindsey also helped brainstorm ideas for the Challenges and developed questions to help the reader actively engage with the material. Their assistance in bringing this work to life cannot be underestimated; they captured the essence of what it is to face the challenges of being an RBT.

We would also like to thank and acknowledge Dan Crafton, Jamiya Eddie, Yamilex Molina, Yamileth Diaz, Madison Williams, Ashton Geiger, Nick Spragg, and Alexandra Manresa for their contributions in focus groups that were designed to evaluate the material.

Disclaimer

This book does not represent an official statement by the Behavior Analyst Certification Board or any other behavior analysis organization. This text cannot be relied on as the only interpretation of the meaning of the RBT Ethics Code or the application of the Code to particular situations. Each RBT, BCBA, supervisor, or relevant agency must interpret and apply the Code as it believes proper, given all of the circumstances.

The *Challenges* used in this book are based on questions sent to ABAEthicsHotline.com as well as from RBTs who have been working in the field for a number of years. Specific cases have been disguised to protect identities.

Part

One

Background for Ethics for Registered Behavior Technicians™

1

How We Got Here

In 2014, the Behavior Analysis Certification Board (BACB) announced a new credential for behavior technicians, the Registered Behavior Technician (RBT). The RBT is a paraprofessional entry-level behavioral technician who practices under the close, ongoing supervision of a Board Certified Assistant Behavior Analyst (BCaBA), Board Certified Behavior Analyst (BCBA), or Board Certified Behavior Analyst-Doctoral (BCBA-D). RBTs play a key role in the direct implementation of behavior analytic services, and they work with individuals with diagnoses such as autism spectrum disorder (ASD), developmental delays, and mental health issues. In January 2016, the BACB received National Commission for Certifying Agencies (NCCA) accreditation for the RBT credential. Clearly, the standards for behavior technicians have come a long way since the early days of behavior analysis that were scarred by the abuse and mistreatment of clients.

THE SUNLAND MIAMI SCANDAL[1]

The Sunland Training Center in Miami, a residential facility for several hundred disabled clients, became "ground zero" for an

1 For the complete history of this incident, please see Chapter 1, "How We Got Here," in *Ethics for Behavior Analysts, 3rd edition*, published in 2016.

abuse investigation that rocked the state of Florida in 1972. After a report of abuse from a parent of a client in April 1971, the Florida Division of Mental Retardation (now the Agency for Persons with Disabilities) and the Dade County attorney's office began an intensive investigation of resident abuse. The director of the State Health and Rehabilitative Services (HRS) Division of Retardation formed a nine-member Blue Ribbon Panel to make recommendations on what to do next in terms of treatment and protecting residential clients from harm. There was very little applied research available at this time. The *Journal of Applied Behavior Analysis*, the professional journal of behavior analysis, had first been published only in 1968, so there was very little research that existed on the application of behavior principles. Further, there was no code of ethics for behavioral researchers or practitioners at this time.

RECOMMENDATIONS OF THE BLUE RIBBON COMMITTEE

The Blue Ribbon Committee took on itself the additional responsibility of making recommendations to prevent any future systematic abuses in the name of behavior modification in the state of Florida. These included strong support for a statewide advocacy program in which staff members would be allowed to make unannounced visits to residential institutions and to collect information from key personnel as well as residents, parents, staff, and concerned citizens. In addition, the committee recommended professional peer review of all behavior programs to ensure that treatment was derived from the literature and that no procedures would be used that were considered "experimental."

FOLLOW-UP

The Florida Association for Retarded Children (now the Association for Retarded Citizens of Florida) took up the cause of humane treatment and ultimately endorsed the notion of supporting data-based behavioral treatment, using strict guidelines, under close supervision by properly trained professionals. The Division of Retardation instituted reforms, including setting up both statewide and local peer review committees for behavior modification programming in facilities throughout Florida.

The Florida Statewide Peer Review Committee for Behavior Modification (PRC) then established a set of guidelines for the use of behavioral procedures, which were subsequently adopted by the National Association for Retarded Citizens (MR Research, 1976) and by the Florida Division of Retardation. The state-funded PRC proceeded to make visits to institutions around the state over the next several years educating staff members about the guidelines and making recommendations for more ethical treatment. The PRC, in conjunction with Florida Association for Behavior Analysis (FABA) (founded in 1980), began the process of certifying behavior analysts via a testing program sponsored by the Division of Retardation. In 1988, the FABA membership adopted the FABA Code of Ethics, the first state association to do so.

Ethics is concerned primarily with the edict to "do no harm." In the Florida case, we saw how great harm could be done by well-meaning people and that when appropriate, comprehensive strategies were adopted, abuse was prevented.

It is the purpose of this volume to try to elucidate the current Behavior Analyst Certification Board RBT Ethics Code to assist registered behavior technicians in making the right choices on a daily basis.

2

Core Ethical Principles for Behavior Analysts Including RBTs

Behavior analysts and registered behavior technicians are part of a culture of caring individuals who seek to improve the lives of others. They carry with them a set of core ethical values that are derived from thousands of years of compassionate practices. (The term *ethics* comes from the Greek word *ethos*, meaning moral character.) It is the purpose of this volume to focus on practical ethics for RBTs, and we first need to discuss some basic moral principles that underlie our culture at large.

In 1998, in their book *Ethics in Psychology*, Koocher and Keith-Spiegel outlined nine ethical principles for psychologists. These principles can be applied to ethics in many areas, including clinical and counseling psychology, the teaching of children, and even the training of animals.

1. DOING NO HARM

The phrase "Do no harm" is typically referred to as appearing in the Hippocratic oath that is taken by physicians. Although no behavior analyst would knowingly do harm, it can come in subtle forms that need to be attended to carefully. One obvious example is that of a behavior analyst who is practicing outside his or her area of expertise (RBT Codes 3.03, 3.04, and 3.05).

2. RESPECTING AUTONOMY

To respect one's autonomy means to promote his or her independence or self-sufficiency. Clearly, the basic procedures of behavior analysis are designed to do just this: prompting, shaping, chaining, and fading and the use of conditioned reinforcers, token economies, and supportive environments are all designed to change behavior in such a way that the person can ultimately deliver his or her own reinforcers rather than depending on a mediator.

3. BENEFITING OTHERS

It almost goes without saying that the primary role of behavior analysts is to benefit others in whatever setting or situation they may work. This principle can often put the behavior analyst at odds with other professionals and requires frequent checks on "who is the client?" in any given situation.

4. BEING JUST

This principle is very basic and is directly derived from the "Golden Rule." Being just means that you should treat others as you would like to be treated. A further refinement of this rule might ask, "How would I like my mother or my child to be treated in similar circumstances?" Questions of just treatment arise often in behavior analysis because there is often so little known about the origins of a particular behavior, and functional relationships often assumed are yet to be determined.

5. BEING FAITHFUL

Well-respected professionals attain their reputation based on the trust placed in them by others. Those who are loyal, trustworthy, and honest (RBT Code 1.03) are sought out as dependable and reliable sources of wise counsel and effective, ethical treatment.

Being truthful and honest with clients, colleagues, and administrators provides the basis for long-term relationships that make for a successful career.

6. ACCORDING DIGNITY

Many of the clients we serve are not able to effectively represent themselves. They may be nonverbal or simply unable to get someone to listen to them. If their wishes are unknown and they are unable to make choices, they may become depressed and present behavior problems that come to the attention of a behavior analyst. Although it is not a "behavioral" term, low self-esteem seems to capture the essence of a person who has not been afforded dignity. As behavior analysts, our job is to make sure that every client is treated with dignity and respect. Behaviorally, this means that we would work with clients on acquisition skills to make sure that they are able to voice or signal their needs to those around them. These individuals should be given choices throughout the day and allowed to exercise their preferences for food, clothing, roommate, activities, and living conditions (RBT Codes 2.01 and 2.02). Other more subtle ways of according dignity involve the language we use to talk to or about clients. If you want to know how Bertha feels about her treatment plan, you could ask the staff or family, or you could ask Bertha herself. Clients should be addressed by name in a friendly fashion using eye contact and a pleasant smile the kind of treatment you expect when you go to a doctor's or dentist's office.

7. TREATING OTHERS WITH CARING AND COMPASSION

Many of the previous ethical principles relate to this ethical principle. If, as a behavior analyst, you respect the autonomy of clients, work to benefit them, and devise programs that accord them dignity, you will automatically be treating clients with care and compassion. This value also suggests not only that clients be given choices but also that interpersonal relationships should demonstrate sympathy and concern.

8. PURSUIT OF EXCELLENCE

Behavior analysis is a rapidly growing field. RBTs need to stay current with new developments as well as constantly updated BACB rules and regulations that are posted in the BACB Newsletter. Excellence in this profession means being at least aware of the latest research in the field, and if you are an RBT, it means working with your BCBA supervisor to ensure that your team is using the most up-to-date methods and procedures in your practice of behavior analysis. Ideally, RBTs would subscribe to one of the key journals in the field and attend state association meetings if at all possible.

9. ACCEPTING ACCOUNTABILITY

RBTs have a tremendous responsibility in providing treatment according to the behavior plan that has been generated by the BCBA supervisor. Treatment fidelity means following the plan exactly as you were trained to do and as it is written. Taking data according to the protocol provided is another part of treatment fidelity and is essential for your accountability.

RBTs do not begin their ethical training in college; it begins long before that. Psychologists have established that ethical standards are likely well set by the time a child ventures into junior high school. Those morals set in childhood may conflict with what it means to be a professional. It is for these reasons that the RBT Ethics Code has been developed for behavior analysts. It is our hope that by reviewing these principles and examining the RBT Code carefully, RBTs will come to see the value in adopting a set of responsible behaviors that will advance the profession and provide respect to the important field of behavior analysis.

3

A *Virtual* Bill of Rights for RBTs

PREAMBLE

Registered Behavior Technicians are on the frontline of treatment. This is especially true when working with children diagnosed with autism spectrum disorder. When working with children with ASD, RBTs have the very difficult job of dealing with deep-seated language deficits, dysfunctional social skills, and severe behavior disorders. While contending with these challenging behaviors, they are often treated badly by parents who are in disagreement with the behavior plan or the company that employs the RBT. These parents might take their dissatisfaction out on the person they see the most often—the therapist. In some cases, the working conditions that RBTs are subjected to are unclean, unhealthy, and dangerous. At the same time, the supervision they receive may stray far from the ideal and range from minimal at best to negligent at worst.[1] None of this should be happening to dedicated, hard-working, and caring individuals who represent our field to the world on a daily basis.

RBTs should have their own *Bill of Rights* to protect them, and, as a matter of fact, they do. This implicit charter is hiding in plain

1 We should point out that the majority of supervisors you will encounter are kind, honest, diligent, and ethical. They strive to train supervisees and RBTs to become better, more ethical behavior analysts and are committed to their welfare and as well as their professional development.

> *"Your supervisor is obliged to tell you the truth and deal with you honestly."*

sight and has been since 2016 when the *Professional and Ethical Compliance Code for Behavior Analysts* went into effect. Although these rights have not been codified, more than a dozen sections of the Compliance Code currently lay out the basic rights to which RBTs are entitled. What follows is an unofficial[2] enumeration, explanation, and interpretation of those rights as derived from the BACB Code of Ethics.

1.04 Integrity

(a) "Behavior analysts are truthful and honest." This item can be interpreted to mean that your supervisor is obliged to tell you the truth and deal with you honestly. If your client is unhappy with your work and brings this to your supervisor, she should not sugarcoat the information or "forget" to tell you; she should give it to you straight.

1.07 No Exploitation

Code 1.07 (a) makes clear in no uncertain terms that behavior analysts do *not* exploit persons over whom they have supervisory authority. This means that as an RBT, your supervisor is not allowed to ask you to write behavior programs and then pass them on with his signature as if he wrote them. Other examples of exploitation include asking you to do certain tasks "off the clock" such as cleaning up the playroom at the clinic, promising you more hours of work so you are always available but only scheduling you a few hours per week, having you attend training without pay, or asking

2 We refer to this as "unofficial" in that it has not been ratified by any organized body of behavior analysts—yet!

you to provide a positive review of the agency on the company's website. These are all clear examples of the exploitation that can occur when there is a power differential between the supervisee and supervisor.

4.06 and 4.07 Limiting Conditions for Effective Treatment

These two Code items require the BCBA to: 1) specify the conditions necessary for a behavior program to work, and 2) if the conditions are not appropriate for implementation, to make necessary changes so they will work. Presumably, if the conditions are not corrected, the BCBA will discontinue services. So if you as the direct on-site therapist find that the home environment is not conducive to training the client or if the parents are not willing to participate in parent training, you should report this to the BCBA (in writing). The BCBA is then required to do something about this. Cases are often reported[3] where one or more caregivers in the home will berate or harass the RBT by engaging in name-calling, cursing, or even threatening the RBT based on some misguided confusion over treatment goals or procedures. This is absolutely unacceptable, and RBTs do not have to tolerate such abuse.

5.0 Supervision Rights

According to the BACB RBT Supervision Requirements, RBTs must have ongoing supervision for a minimum of 5% of the hours spent providing behavior analytic services per month. The quality of that supervision is questionable in far too many cases where the power differential between BA-level RBTs and master's or PhD-level BCBAs makes any form of effective remediation unlikely. Understanding their specific rights to quality supervision may

3 Through the ABAEthicsHotline.com site run by the first author.

help RBTs make their case. As an RBT, you have a right to quality supervision.

Code 5.0 Behavior Analysts as Supervisors

The key words pertaining to supervisors in this Code item are, "they must take full responsibility for all facets" of supervision. We take "all facets" to include accepting clients that are treatable given the talents and resources of the ABA team, determining that the environment is appropriate for treatment, preparing the teachers or caregivers for their part in the treatment-delivery process, developing a usable data-collection methodology and a behavior plan that is feasible given the resources available, overseeing the arc of treatment from assessment to discharge, and protecting both the client and RBT from harm throughout the process. If any aspect of this entire enterprise is faulty or malfunctioning, it is up to the supervisor to step up and take responsibility.

> *"RBTs are entitled to a competent supervisor."*

5.01 Supervisory Competence

RBTs are entitled to a *competent* supervisor. This is defined by Code 1.02, which says the supervisor should provide services within the boundaries of competence as defined by their "education, training, and supervised experience." For example, if the supervisor assigns you (an RBT) a case involving "pica" or Prader-Willi Syndrome, you would assume that your supervisor had specific training and experience in dealing with these two rather low-probability behavior disorders. It could be awkward to ask about this, but when your supervisor presents you with the behavior plan, you should feel comfortable asking, "This is totally new to me; can you show me how to do this?" Then, you should feel free to judge the competence of your supervisor based on the clarity of the demonstration, her fluency with the procedures involved, and her ability to answer any questions that you might have. You should feel thoroughly comfortable with taking on the case after observing your supervisor model the procedures. If you are not comfortable or have any reservations, it may be that your supervisor is really not competent with cases like this or not skilled at teaching the procedures. In another situation where parents are resisting some aspect of the behavior protocol and you go to your supervisor for help, if he says, "Just take care of it," you could say, "Could we role-play that interaction? I'm not exactly sure how to handle this, and these parents are quite adamant." And again, you will be able to judge your supervisor's competence by his ability to teach you the details of the protocol as he role-plays the part of the troublesome dad.

> *"RBTs are entitled to a supervisor who is not overworked."*

5.02 Supervisory Volume

RBTs are entitled to a supervisor who is not overworked. This would be a supervisor that has not taken on more clients and supervisees than can be *effectively* supervised. A BCBA supervisor who is abiding by Code 5.02 will not allow themselves to be pressed into taking an excessive number of cases that will inevitably lead to less supervision time for the RBTs because with less supervision time, there invariably comes lower-quality monitoring, feedback, and training. This strain on a supervisor's time directly impacts the quality of service to the clients. Similarly, when faced with the necessity of using shortcuts that are unethical and sometimes illegal in order to handle excessive volume, the quality of the supervisor's work is impacted. One very tangible outcome of supervisors having too many supervisees is that RBTs and RBT trainees may not receive the necessary supervision hours required by the Board for their certification. This has serious implications for the professional growth and development of supervisees.

When applying for a position at a company, it is important for RBTs to interview with (in addition to the recruiter) the person who will be their supervisor. It is in this interaction that you can ask about the supervisor's model of supervision and how the supervisor works with RBTs. You should also ask about the size of their caseload and if they expect it to expand any time in the near future.

> *"RBTs are entitled to a supervisor who only assigns tasks that are feasible."*

5.03 Supervisory Delegation

RBTs are entitled to a supervisor who only assigns tasks that are *feasible* for someone who is working an entry-level position with limited training and experience. It is the responsibility of RBTs to hold their supervisors in check and not accept duties that are over their heads or unreasonable given the circumstances. This is where Code 5.03 can help if you find yourself being assigned tasks where you do not have the necessary skills "to perform competently, ethically, and safely." Note that Code 5.03 is complementary with RBT Ethics Code 3.03, so all you need to do is ask if this request or requirement meets Code item 3.03. You might say, for example, "I'm not comfortable developing a functional assessment on my own, and I don't want to violate my RBT Ethics Code 3.03; can you work with me on this?"

> *"RBTs are entitled to receive supervision and training which is effective."*

5.04 Designing Effective Supervision and Training

RBTs are entitled to *receive* supervision and training that is effective. Effectiveness is determined by how well the RBT or other supervisee performs following the training. You should be able to acquire the skills presented fairly quickly and put them to immediate use since the training has been developed by your experienced, well-trained behavior analyst supervisor who is competent in developing task analyses and knows how to use behavioral techniques such as forward and backward chaining, shaping, and other strategies such as behavioral skills training (BST), TAG Teaching, and so on.

Included in this code item is that the content of the training should be behavior-analytic and meet your requirements for supervision hours as specified by the BACB.

> *"RBTs are entitled to receive effective supervision and training."*

5.05 Communication of Supervision Conditions

As an RBT you are entitled to "a clear written description of the purpose, requirements, evaluation criteria, conditions, and terms of supervision prior to the onset of the supervision." Basically, according to Code 5.05, RBTs are *entitled* to receive effective supervision and training as required of all supervisors. If you have not received such a written description, which might also be called a *supervision contract* or *supervision agreement*, you have a right to ask for one. Once you have it in hand, look it over carefully to make sure that you understand each section.

The *purpose* should specify the reason that you are receiving supervision; the requirements section should cover all aspects of the supervisee/RBT position from the number of hours that you will be working, the types of clients you will be working with in your job, the way that you will record your hours, the consequences for missing work, and so on.

Under *evaluation criteria*, your supervisor should make clear how you will be evaluated including how often and under what conditions you will be observed, what behaviors she will be observing, what rating system or data recording will be used, and how you will receive feedback resulting from these observations.

Next, your supervision contract should specify the *conditions under which you are expected to work*, that is, will it be an in-home or clinic or possibly a classroom setting; will you be expected to carry out emergency procedures and, if the latter, the type of training you will receive should be specified. There should be a clear explanation of conditions under which your supervisor will and will not sign the form to document your hours; supervisors are known to withhold their signature for unspecified reasons, so be certain that this sort of situation is thoroughly explained and that you fully understand the implications.

> *"Your capability as a technician should become better over time as a result of how your supervisor supports your work with clients."*

Finally, in the *terms of supervision* section, this will provide you with conditions included in the contract and will describe what a breach of contract would involve. In addition, this section should specify the consequences for such a breach and the consequences if you should drop out before the contract ends.

5.06 Providing Feedback to Supervisees

As an RBT, you are *entitled* by this Code to "feedback and reinforcement systems" developed and implemented by your supervisor. These systems work to actually improve your performance in real time. Feedback might include verbal, written, or graphic feedback, and reinforcement *systems* could include some sort of achievement checklist that leads to longer-term rewards like access to company rewards, special privileges, or advancement within the agency. This is an interesting guarantee since it is not based on topography of behavior-change systems (e.g.,

> *"BCBAs should serve as role models for ethical conduct."*

you will receive two hours of BST per week) but rather the *outcome*; that is, your capability as a technician should become better over time as a result of how your supervisor supports your work with clients. There is a presumption here that, as mentioned earlier, your supervisor has given you a set of objective standards for each type of therapy for which you are involved and that the feedback is given in a timely fashion so that you can make corrections if necessary. Feedback will help you know that what you are doing is worthy and appreciated.

7.01 Right to Work in an Ethical Environment

This very short Code item carries a great deal of meaning to RBTs, "Behavior analysts promote an ethical culture in their work environments and make others aware of this Code." There are several steps that the behavior analysts in your organization can take to make sure that you are working in an ethical culture.

1. BCBAs should serve as role models for ethical conduct. This includes how they handle themselves with clients, how they engage with colleagues, and most especially how they treat their supervisees. Not showing up for supervision, making demeaning or condescending comments about supervisees in meetings, and asking RBTs to backdate supervision forms are all examples of unethical conduct that should not occur in an *ethical culture*.
2. BCBAs should discuss ethics during supervision and training sessions as well as in conversations, meetings, and company newsletters. Ethical practices should be highlighted on a regular basis and RBTs should be given an opportunity to express any ethical concerns that they have during one-to-one as well as group sessions.
3. Behavior analyst owners of companies should establish an ethics officer and ethics committee (in larger organizations) that will offer ongoing ethics training, bring in ethics

speakers, and handle ethics complaints on a confidential basis.

4. Behavior analyst supervisors should visibly reinforce ethical behavior and deal quickly and appropriately with unethical conduct in the work environment. There is nothing that reduces morale more than seeing someone, who is perhaps a favorite employee, getting away with violating the rules and ethical guidelines.

SUMMARY

We urge all RBTs to carefully examine their rights as described previously and incorporate them into regular conversations with their supervisors as well as other RBTs. Our profession can only grow strong and vital if everyone respects the rights of those on the front line of treatment.

Part

Two

Introducing the RBT® Ethics Code

4

Section 1—Responsible Conduct Codes 1.01–1.13

The purpose of this section of the RBT Ethics Code is to lay out the basic expectations of appropriate conduct by RBTs in their day-to-day interactions with their clients, colleagues, supervisors, and other professionals. We expect you to know the basic principles of behavior analysis and to defend and promote those principles as you interact with all of these individuals throughout the day (Code 1.01). This is no small feat since challenges can come at any time and in any size. Such challenges range from a parent asking you to implement an exotic-sounding treatment they have read about on the internet to a teacher requesting your assistance with implementing one of the latest fads that regularly sweep through elementary school districts. Some of our basic principles involve behavior-analytic methods that have been developed over the past 50 years. Most of these methods have been published in studies that are based on solid research methodology and have been published in the *Journal of Applied Behavior Analysis* and more recently in *Behavior Analysis in Practice*. It would be very useful for you to know these well enough to discuss them with those that you run into throughout the day.

You are expected to be well versed in the entire code and to be able to quickly identify appropriate and inappropriate behaviors that you might need to exhibit or avoid (Code 1.02). You can think of the code as consisting of rules that you need to abide by, just like the rules you need to follow when driving. Driving "rules" are posted as road signs, and claiming ignorance about them will not keep you from getting a ticket. *Slow Down, Yield, Stop, No Right Turn on Red* are rules of the road for a fundamental reason; they keep you and the other drivers on the road safe. Knowing and following our code will keep you safe from criticism and censure and your clients safe from harm.

It does not seem like too high a bar to ask RBTs to be truthful and honest (Code 1.03) and expect this conduct from others. However, there is a colossal amount of dishonesty in the world today. We are inundated by misleading advertising and scam robocalls that attempt to deceive us at every turn. We are faced with attempts to lure us into buying cheap defective products or deliver our hard-earned savings to a stranger to help a stranded relative. We hope RBTs will not fall prey to such deceptive ploys and that in your dealings with your clients, supervisors, and agencies, you will set a standard of being forthright and honest. Closely associated with this is a desire for all RBTs to operate within the boundaries of the law and follow the legal codes of their community (Code 1.04). If you have an ethical conflict with a policy of your company, our code recommends that you bring it directly to your supervisor (Code 1.05) for a quick resolution. Be sure to document any ethical conflicts that you bring to your supervisor in writing. For example, after speaking directly to your supervisor about a concern, you might send an email along the lines of, "Thank you for speaking with me today. To summarize our conversation . . . "

RBTs work in close concert with clients and their families, and while it may be tempting to be drawn into the client's personal circle of friends, this is a serious mistake. Our code describes this as a multiple relationship, which is to be avoided under all circumstances. (This is detailed in Chapter 4, Code 1.06.) One sad outcome of a multiple relationship occurs when a "friendship" escalates to a sexual relationship. This is most often totally destructive to all parties concerned (Code 1.07). In the same vein are other personal problems that you could have in your adult life that can lead to depression, anxiety, and possibly the misuse of alcohol and drugs. Our code advises that if you have any of these problems that could affect your duties and responsibilities, you seek help immediately (Code 1.08).

For many RBTs, their new position as a "behavior tech" in a company will be their first serious, professional position. The job of the RBT is much different than waiting tables or flipping burgers. As a professional, you are expected to carefully consider any commitments you make and to make sure that you are able to follow through on each of them to the best of your ability (Code 1.09). This includes signing contracts for employment that are legally binding.

It is easy to get excited by the outcomes and potential for behavior analysis, especially if you are working closely with child clients who might initially have no social skills, no language, and few self-care skills. With these children, in just a few months, you may start to see amazing progress, including first words, direct eye contact, and elementary social play with other children. However, Code 1.10 cautions against making false or exaggerated statements that misrepresent our field or give false hope to parents and other caregivers.

When you are applying for a job in behavior analysis, it is important that you be truthful and accurate in your representations to potential employers and that you keep them up to date as to your certification status (Code 1.11). Somewhat related to this is your need to always obtain permission to use copyrighted or trademarked material (Code 1.12).

Finally, in Section 1, our code emphasizes that you must work closely with your BACB supervisor to try to resolve any issues you may have informally (Code 1.13). The exception to this is if it involves a client safety issue. In this case, it may be necessary to involve other legal authorities such as Child Protective Services.

For the questions that follow, select the *best* answer to the question.

1.01 RBTs UPHOLD AND PROMOTE THE VALUES AND CORE PRINCIPLES OF BEHAVIOR ANALYSIS

> "The values of behavior analysis include a commitment to the study of socially significant, individual human behavior and to a methodology for changing that behavior to the betterment of the individual and society."

Quick Take

This first Code item requires all RBTs to confirm their commitment to the core ethical values described in Chapter 2, the science of behavior, and to advocate for the basic principles of behavior analysis when appropriate. The values of behavior analysis include a commitment to the study of socially significant, individual human behavior and to a methodology for changing that behavior to the betterment of the individual and society. Behavior analysis is widely recognized as the foremost science of human behavior and relies on applied research to help our clients.

Basic principles of behavior include positive and negative reinforcement, punishment, conditioned and unconditioned reinforcers, and stimulus control. Extinction of responses that are maintained by a known reinforcer is a principle embedded in many behavior programs, as is the concept of the motivating operation.

CHALLENGE 1: You are driving to work, listening to a podcast about autism, and hear the host say, "We all know that ABA should not be used with children; it is way too aversive. I mean, they still use corporal punishment."

RBT RESPONSE: You could speak with your supervisor about the podcast when you get to work and discuss whether you should send an email to the host and provide him with research and feedback about behavior analysis. You could also ask your supervisor if she would like to review what you have written or add in their feedback as well.

COMMENTARY: This is a good way to handle a situation like this. As an RBT, it is important to advocate for this field. It is important to disseminate accurate research, and discussing an issue like this with your supervisor before contacting the podcaster is the best option. Some supervisors would ask that you do this as an individual and that you not identify the agency.

CHALLENGE 2: You arrive at a client's home to a visibly angry parent. He informs you that his son had a bad day at school and therefore will not be allowed to play with any of his toys (thus restricting access to all previously identified reinforcers).

WHAT NOT TO DO: You tell the father, "Okay, I guess we will just have to figure out something else to do today." Your programs depend on being able to offer a break only during reinforcement periods.

WHAT *TO* DO: Inform the father that in order for you to conduct therapy, you must be able to deliver effective reinforcers to build new skills. Without access to reinforcers, you will not be able to provide the necessary motivation for treatment. You should also inquire more about the behaviors that occurred at school and let the father know you can speak to your supervisor and see if she has any idea of how to help address it.

COMMENTARY: It is not uncommon to run into situations where the programs you need to implement will conflict with a parent's disciplinary methods. As the RBT, it is your job to try to educate the parent on the principles of reinforcement. You should convey to the parent that the client isn't just "playing" but earned the reinforcement through his work on the treatment plan. It might be a good idea to ask the father what you can use instead of toys, or you might need to contact your supervisor about the situation.

CHALLEGE 3: It is the first day working with Logan Ferguson, who reportedly engages in mild disruptive behavior, non-compliance, and threatening self-injurious behavior (SIB) (remember that we have changed names to protect identities throughout the book). Your task is to record the normal interactions of the family with Logan to establish a baseline and collect ABC (Antecedent Behavior Consequence) data. Mom approaches you after 30 minutes or so and says, "I thought you were here to treat these annoying problems; you're just watching us and playing on your iPad. I'm going to call your supervisor."

RBT RESPONSE: "I'm sorry, Mrs. Ferguson. My supervisor should have explained that before we can begin treatment, we need to have a good idea of how Logan normally interacts with you and other family members. This is our baseline. We also need to know how severe the behaviors are and how often they occur. I am collecting data on this iPad; this is how I do my job. Let me show you what I have so far . . . "

COMMENTARY: This RBT did a great job explaining one of the bedrock methods of our field, which is direct observation and data collection. She carefully explained that without a baseline, we really don't know where to start treatment and will not be able to make comparisons with any treatment effects that will follow.

> "Our primary commitment is to the study of learned behaviors."

More Details

We take seriously the seven dimensions of ABA as outlined by Baer, Wolf, and Risley (1968). These are our guiding principles: our field is applied, behavioral, analytic, technological, relevant to our conceptual system, effective, and produces behavior change that proves to be durable over time and across settings (generality). Our primary commitment is to the study of learned behaviors (those acquired through operant conditioning) and the use of positive reinforcement strategies to effect change. Single-case designs with clear experimental control provide the empirical evidence that is the foundation of behavior analysis.

Even more basically, you can describe behavior analysis as a branch of science in which we emphasize the importance of direct observation of behavior: systematic, reliable data collection that then allows the *prediction* of behavior. When prediction is possible, the next step is to find ways to change behavior if behavior change is needed for the individual to become more independent, find relief from SIB, or cause less harm to others. The science of behavior is based on determinism.

In summary, behavior analysis revolves around the concept of the operant (learned behavior), the importance of the environment in determining whether a behavior will occur (stimulus control), and the central principle that consequences matter. In fact, almost all behavior is shaped by consequences, and this produces a history of reinforcement for the individual that determines how they will conduct themselves day to day.

Please Note: *While some of the choices in the multiple-choice response options that follow may seem humorous, sarcastic, and even somewhat "edgy"; however, we are assured that they have been overheard in conversations among RBTs in a variety of settings and circumstances.*

Code 1.01 Test Yourself: Multiple-Choice Questions

1. A parent informed you that her child had just been put on a gluten-free/casein-free diet and that all edibles used during therapy needed to follow the diet. The parent then asked you to work on allowing the child to play with her food because it's going to "integrate" the child

with the food and eating process. How should you respond?

a. "Absolutely; I think that sounds like a great idea."
b. "Unfortunately, those are not considered evidence-based practices in ABA, and it would be unethical for me to implement those, but I can talk to my supervisor if you would like to work on incorporating more foods into her diet."
c. "Are you sure? 'Playing with food' doesn't sound very appetizing to me."
d. "I am not sure your child will learn to eat properly if we let her play with food."

2. When you were working with your client, a child who engages in self-injurious behavior, another therapist (not an RBT) who also works with the client told you that he wanted to start putting the child into a swing every time the SIB occurs. His theory was that this will interrupt the synapses and cause the child to relax, thereby eliminating the need for SIB. The therapist told you that when the SIB happens, you should immediately rush her to the swing and push her until the SIB stops. How should you respond?
   a. "Never am I ever going to do that."
   b. "You are only reinforcing the SIB by letting the child swing."
   c. "I am not sure that I will be able to implement that; we have a specific protocol for SIB, but you can contact my supervisor if you would like to discuss it further."
   d. "I think you don't understand how behavior works."
3. You and another RBT were discussing a client who engaged in high levels of aggression. The RBT told you that she was getting frustrated and the protocols weren't working to decrease the aggression. The RBT told you that she accidentally squeezed the client's wrist too hard during a blocking response, and the client immediately stopped.

Since then, the other RBT has been squeezing the client's arm when the child engages in aggression. How should you respond?

a. "That is violating our code of ethics, and you are not upholding the principles of ABA. I will discuss this with our supervisor."
b. "Yes, she is a difficult client, so I can understand getting frustrated."
c. "I'm not sure that is what we are supposed to do when the aggression happens."
d. "Oh, okay, do what you need to survive, I guess."

Code 1.01 Test Yourself: True or False Question

4. The mother of a client you were working with in the home just told you that their dog has been chewing everything in the house. Mom said, "You are a behavior person, so I thought you could help with our dog's bad behavior." The thought crossed your mind that if you give Mom some suggestions to help with the dog, she might go away and you can finish your session. It is okay for you to give her some advice about how to handle her dog.

   True or False?
   True
   False

For correct answers, see Appendix A

FOR FURTHER READING

Baer, D. M., Wolf, M. M., & Risley, T. R. (1968). Some current dimensions of applied behavior analysis. *Journal of Applied Behavior Analysis, 1*, 91–97.

Wallace, M., & Mayer, G. R. (2019). *Principles of Applied Behavior Analysis for Behavior Technicians (BTs) and Other Practitioners.* Cornwall on Hudson: Sloan Publishing.

1.02 RBTs HAVE AN OBLIGATION TO REMAIN FAMILIAR WITH THIS CODE. LACK OF KNOWLEDGE OR UNDERSTANDING OF THIS CODE DOES NOT EXCUSE UNETHICAL CONDUCT

> "'Ignorance will not set you free' is the motto to live by."

Quick Take

Registered Behavior Analysts have an obligation to be familiar with this RBT Ethics Code. Lack of awareness or misunderstanding of a conduct standard is not itself a defense to a charge of unethical conduct.

Familiarity with the ethics Code is essentially *required* of ALL candidates and certificants. "Ignorance will not set you free" is the motto to live by. Behavior analysts who try to use their lack of knowledge of the Code to excuse lapses of judgment in the daily execution of professional responsibilities should be reminded that this is not acceptable. Certificants who reside in states that license behavior analysts are similarly required to be aware of the code of ethics that governs their practice.

CHALLENGE 1: Sally is an RBT who observes Rann, another RBT, incorrectly score data for a client. She asks Rann about what she has seen, and, based on his response, Sally mentions that it is unethical to falsify data. Rann replies that he didn't know there was a code of ethics for RBTs, so he shouldn't be accused of something like this.

RBT RESPONSE: Sally should have mentioned to Rann that it is unethical not to know the code, and it is part of upholding the RBT credential to fully understand the RBT Ethics Code. Sally could have directed Rann to the BACB.com website and suggested that a conversation with his BCBA supervisor is in order since the client's data is not accurate.

CHALLENGE 2: An experienced junior RBT who received her certification in 2016 was asked by a recent certificant about a specific Code item. "If I don't agree with one of our boss's rules, do I need to say something? I really think it's not right to discharge clients just because they have less than 20 hours of behavioral services."

SENIOR RBT RESPONSE: "There is a lot going on around here that's not right; just keep your head down and do your job."

JUNIOR RBT: "But I was reading Code 1.05, and it seems to say that we have to bring conflicts like this to our supervisor's attention and put our concerns in writing."

SENIOR RBT: "What RBT Ethics Code? What are you talking about?"

JUNIOR RBT: "Never mind."

COMMENTARY: This is a perfect example of a more senior-level RBT knowing less about the RBT Code of Ethics than a junior tech. In addition, not knowing about the code is a direct violation of Code 1.02.

> "RBTs are the eyes and ears of behavior analysis and they need to thoroughly understand the Code to keep themselves and others in check."

More Details

Being familiar with the RBT Ethics Code is vital to the practice of behavior analysis since the Ethics Code establishes the rules that we follow to keep our clients safe and our profession honest, effective, and honorable. RBTs are the eyes and ears of behavior analysis, and they need to thoroughly understand the Code to keep themselves and others in check.

Organizations that employ RBTs should have regular, monthly meetings with the RBTs to review Code items and answer questions regarding client treatment plans, professional conduct among staff members, and communications with upper management.

Code 1.02 Test Yourself: Multiple-Choice Questions

1. You are seeking to earn your RBT and are currently working as a behavior technician. You asked an RBT that is currently working at your agency how she earned the 40 hours necessary for the credential. The RBT told you that she completed an online module for the training portion. Looking into the training modules, you noticed that there was only 1 hour of ethics training when you know 3 hours are required. You asked the RBT how she completed the remainder of the ethics hours. The RBT replied with, "Oh, I didn't know we needed that many. I simply reported my hours." How should you respond?
   a. "Well, not knowing the ethical code is unethical. You are not exempt from the code because you were unaware."
   b. "That was smart to just sign it and be done with it."
   c. "I'm sure you have made up for the additional required ethics training since you sat for your exam."
   d. "It's okay; I won't tell anyone."
2. Another RBT from your company is working with a client at a school. This RBT is putting a weighted vest on the client because the teacher asked him to do this when the client engaged in problem behaviors. You have now seen the RBT use this weighted vest with other clients as well. How should you respond to the other RBT?
   a. "I would like to try this, too. Where can I get a weighted vest?"
   b. "I totally understand just trying to make the teacher happy, and I will not say anything about this."
   c. "In Code 1.01, it says as RBTs we are supposed to uphold the principles of behavior analysis, and that means we

don't use non-behavior-analytic procedures. It's in our code to be familiar with that."

d. "I am guessing because you are using this vest, it must be working."

3. As a brand-new RBT, you want to make sure that you are abiding by the code of ethics. However, there are code items that you don't quite understand and aren't sure where to find the information. What should you do?
   a. Just carry on with your therapy sessions and hope that you eventually learn the information by working with clients.
   b. Ask your supervisor to create an ethics-focused meeting where everyone can meet and discuss any BACB updates or ethics situations that have arisen.
   c. Understand that if those code items were important, they would have been on the RBT exam.
   d. Decide that you don't need to understand each code item because you are a moral person and would never do anything wrong.

Code 1.02 Test Yourself: True or False Question

4. While observing another RBT's session, you noticed the client was picked up 30 minutes early by his parents. You saw the other RBT completing the hours sheet, and he billed for the entire session. You mentioned to the RBT that billing for times when therapy did not occur is wrong and violates the RBT Ethics Code. The RBT replied that it was okay to bill for the entire session because he has to clean up after the client leaves. This is ethically acceptable.

   True or False?

   True

   False

For correct answers, see Appendix A

1.03 RBTs ARE TRUTHFUL AND HONEST AND CREATE AN ENVIRONMENT THAT PROMOTES TRUTHFUL AND HONEST BEHAVIOR IN OTHERS. THEY PROMOTE AN ETHICAL CULTURE IN THEIR WORK ENVIRONMENTS AND MAKE OTHERS AWARE OF THIS CODE

> "Promoting an ethical culture means noticing ethical conduct on the part of colleagues and finding ways to encourage those behaviors."

Quick Take

This element requiring RBTs to be truthful and honest, often referred to as *integrity*, represents a foundation for all ethics codes. If you knowingly give misinformation to a client and this is found out later, they will not trust you in the future. The same goes with your supervisor or administration officials. If you provide a distorted version of what happened to a client when you were out in the community or try to deceive your supervisor about your part in an unfortunate incident, they will not hold you in high regard and will not trust you with future responsibilities.

Promoting an ethical culture means noticing ethical conduct on the part of colleagues and finding ways to encourage those behaviors. It also means giving feedback when necessary to try to educate another RBT about the need to follow the RBT Ethics Code at all times.

CHALLENGE 1: Gabe contacted his supervisor late at night and told her that he is having a family emergency and needed to be excused from his sessions for the next two days because he had to go home and be with his family. The supervisor immediately gave him the time off and told him to take as long as he needed. A week later, the supervisor overheard Gabe talking to his work friends.

RBT: "Yeah, I just said I had a family emergency, and she let me out of work."

SUPERVISOR: "I can't believe that you would lie about a family emergency instead of requesting the time off as the employee handbook outlines. Not only are you breaking the rules of the handbook, but you are also violating Code 1.03 and not being truthful and honest."

COMMENTARY: Gabe violated Code 1.03 by lying to the supervisor. It's also important for him to be updated on the RBT Code of Ethics. He should have known that he was not only being unprofessional but was also violating a code item.

CHALLENGE 2: A group of RBTs who are known to be friends outside of work have often boasted about the number of times they have either come into work hung over or high. A few of these RBTs have made a habit of calling in sick because they partied the night before. Another RBT is aware of the behaviors that are occurring by this group and often sees their comments related to this posted on social media.

RBT RESPONSE: You decide that it's not your problem, and it doesn't really affect you, so you keep quiet.

COMMENTARY: Code 1.03 applies to both the group of RBTs that are engaging in these poor behaviors and to the RBT that is aware of it. As the RBT, you should be going to the supervisor and telling him what you know and saw on social media. The supervisor should intervene with the group of RBTs about their work habits. As an RBT, you need to have integrity and be honest with what you know and uphold the code.

CHALLENGE 3: A supervisor heard through the grapevine that one of her RBTs was accepting gifts from a client family. She spoke with the family about this, and they confirmed the rumor, stating, "We thought it was no big deal.

We like giving small tokens of appreciation to anyone who helps our child. We know that some therapists won't accept these small tokens, but Toni does and I'm sure she can use the money." The supervisor then went to the RBT to find out the truth.

RBT: "No, I wouldn't accept gifts; I know that's wrong."

SUPERVISOR: "Are you sure? I spoke to Carl's parents and they told a different story."

RBT: "Well, okay, maybe it happened once, but the parents insisted; they said I was doing such good work with Carl that I deserved a little something for my extra effort."

SUPERVISOR: "Toni, the parents say that they have given you $20 on more than one occasion and that you hinted to them that you were coming up short and sure could use a little extra to repair your car."

RBT: "They said that?"

SUPERVISOR: "They did, and I'm really disappointed in you. I've talked with the clinical director, and we are removing you from Carl's case and cutting your hours for the next month. You clearly violated Code 1.03 by being dishonest with me, and you also violated Code 2.04 by accepting gifts. I am filing a written notice with the director. Since this is your first offense, we will not report you to the Board this time, but if it happens again, we will.

RBT: "I'm so sorry; I guess I didn't realize how important this was. Can I get an extra copy of the Ethics Code to review?"

SUPERVISOR: "Go to BACB.com and type 'ethics' in the search box."

COMMENTARY: An unethical situation can only be made worse by trying to cover it up. Toni violated two different code items in this challenge. She violated Code 1.03 by lying to her supervisor about accepting the gifts. It's possible that if the BCBA hadn't pushed for an answer, she would have continued accepting the gifts while being dishonest about it. When a violation has been brought to your attention, it is best to be forthright so that you can begin the necessary steps to remedy the situation.

> "Tests of your integrity can come flying at you nearly every week."

More Details

"Integrity is doing the right thing even if no one is looking" is often quoted as a test of one's character, and it is why integrity is one of the first items in the RBT Ethics Code. Integrity is considered a foundation of a good person, one who can be trusted under all circumstances to make tough decisions and tell the truth even if it is not in their best interest. Tests of your integrity can come flying at you nearly every week from clients, colleagues, and even your company. A client may ask you to fudge the data a little so they can receive more services. Saying "No" could make you look like a mean, heartless person, but doing so would be wrong, so wrong that it could be fraudulent. An RBT colleague may offer you drugs at a weekend party at the beach. If you accept, you'll be one of the gang, and if you refuse, you could be accused of being a chicken or loser. In another example, your company could tell you to spread the word to clients that insurance requirements are changing and they will need to increase their hours to 20 per week. You know this is not true since you were sitting in the back of the room when a senior associate suggested this strategy to increase the company's bottom line. In all these cases, you will be tested to see if you can come up with a way to refuse this pressure and stay in the game. Learning to push back is one clear way to maintain your integrity.

Code 1.03 Test Yourself: Multiple-Choice Questions

1. As an RBT who is working with a new client, you are experiencing some difficulties with the client's problem

behaviors. The supervisor asked you if the sessions were running okay because the data indicate the client is not making progress. How should you respond?
   a. "Nope, everything is fine, and we are doing great."
   b. "To be honest, I could really use some more training and supervision because I am having some problems."
   c. "Well, actually, the therapists that were training me didn't do a good job and didn't explain much of anything."
   d. "This client doesn't like me, and I don't think I should be working with her."
2. You and another RBT are leaving a session that ended 30 minutes early, but the other RBT is still going to bill for the full length of the session. The RBT tells you, "It's okay; as long as you bill for it, too, we won't get in trouble." How should you respond?
   a. Ignore the other RBT and bill for the time the session actually ended.
   b. Tell the other RBT that you are going to bill for the time the session ended and talk to the supervisor about the over-billing because the other RBT is violating the code of ethics.
   c. Say, "That's a great idea, I'm short this week and need all the hours I can get."
   d. Smile and nod at the RBT so she doesn't get mad, but bill for the accurate time.
3. An RBT who works with you was late getting to a session. The RBT let your supervisor know, but she told him it was because her car wouldn't start. In reality, the car was fine and she overslept. This will be the third time this week that the RBT overslept. She explained this to you because you had to cover her session again. How should you respond?
   a. Tell her, "It's okay. I understand; we are all tired."
   b. Start complaining about how early the session times start and that they should start later so everyone can sleep in.

c. Say, "It's none of my business."
d. Explain to her that she is actually violating the code by lying to the supervisor, and if she doesn't tell him the truth, you will have to.

4. When a senior RBT was training you to work with a client, she said, "Every once in a while, this mother will buy you things or put things in your bag without your knowledge, but they are never very expensive." When you asked if the RBT returned the items to the mother, the RBT said, "It's okay to accept these things because they are small." You began accepting the small surprises that the client's mother put in your bag. Your supervisor found out, and you told her the senior RBT told you this was okay. The senior RBT denies that any of this ever happened. How should you respond?
   a. Quit the job because they are being unfair.
   b. Stand up for what is right. Tell the supervisor the senior RBT is lying, and that you wish to be ethical and uphold Code 1.03 and plan to be honest.
   c. Tell your supervisor that you must have misunderstood the senior RBT, and that you wish to be ethical and uphold Code 1.03 and plan to be honest.
   d. Write an email to the whole company about how the senior RBT is lying.

Code 1.03 Test Yourself: True or False Question

5. While you were on your way to your client's school for his session, your supervisor called and asked you to stop by the clinic and pick up something for the client's new programs. You were running late, and when you got to the school, you realized you forgot to bring the items. When your supervisor asked you if you brought the items for the client's program, you said, "I looked everywhere,

but I couldn't find them. Maybe someone else picked them up." This response was a violation of the code.

True or False?

True

False

For correct answers, see Appendix A

1.04 RBTs ACT IN A WAY THAT CONFORMS TO THE LEGAL AND ETHICAL CODES OF THE PROFESSIONAL AND SOCIAL COMMUNITIES WHERE THEY ARE MEMBERS. THEY DO NOT LEAD OTHERS TO ENGAGE IN FRAUDULENT, ILLEGAL, OR UNETHICAL CONDUCT

> "*Fraudulent conduct* refers to intentional false billing of hours to an insurance company or Medicaid."

Quick Take

This Code item consists of two parts. The first part makes it clear that RBTs are expected to abide by the laws in their community and their state, and the second brings up a related issue; that is, RBTs should not be encouraging any illegal or unethical conduct. The term "*Fraudulent conduct*" refers primarily to intentional false billing of hours to an insurance company or Medicaid. Making a simple clerical error that you catch and correct by bringing it to the attention of your supervisor would not be considered fraud, but regularly billing for service hours not provided would be a fraudulent practice. Encouraging other employees in an ABA company to bill for services not provided is also unethical under this Code element. Claiming that you had passed the RBT Competency Assessment when you had not would be considered a misrepresentation or *deceitful* and therefore would also be a form of fraud.

CHALLENGE 1: At a party, an RBT noticed there were drugs present. The RBT's colleagues from work were telling him,

"It's okay; try some; no one will find out." The RBT knew that there was a no-drugs policy at his clinic and random drug tests were administered.

RBT RESPONSE: "No, I can't do that. It's against the law and I don't want to risk losing my certification, or my job, or getting arrested."

COMMENTARY: This RBT was absolutely correct in refusing to participate. Even if your company does not have a drug policy or test for drugs, participating in illegal drug activity violates the law, and this is a violation of the code. It is important to remember that you live in a community with laws and those laws have to be upheld along with the code.

CHALLENGE 2: You just started working with a new client at your company. While in training, you were told that the client naps during part of her school day and during that time, you should sit in the room with her. You asked how to bill during the time the client was sleeping, and the lead tech said, "Just bill insurance as though the client was engaged."

RBT RESPONSE: "Does the compliance officer know she naps during that time? I don't feel comfortable billing while I am not providing treatment. I will have to go check with the BCBA."

COMMENTARY: The lead tech should have been aware of the potential billing fraud that can occur when turning in an hours sheet for a client that is sleeping. That RBT should not have passed on incorrect information, and the new RBT was correct in questioning this and proceeding to check in with the BCBA.

CHALLENGE 3: "I completed the 40-hour training and went to the agency to take the oral exam. My supervisor began by signing off on parts of the competency exam that she believed were too simple to discuss. She would ask if I knew the definition of something on the task list. If I did not know the definition, she would explain what it was and then sign off. If I said I did know the definition, she would sign off on the tasks without an explanation from me. Then my supervisor told me I was supposed to practice some of the items on the Task List with a client. She decided the timing for me to do this wasn't convenient, so she signed off on the completion of the tasks anyway. I was very uncomfortable with this. It felt wrong, but this BCBA was going to be my new supervisor."

RBT ALTERNATIVE RESPONSE: After the supervisor started signing off on incomplete or incorrect tasks: "Ms. Russell, I really don't feel comfortable with this. Maybe I should just stop here and come back another day."

COMMENTARY: Although we expect all supervisors to act ethically, this unfortunately is not always the case. You may not have control over a supervisor's unethical behavior, but you can do your part to ensure that it does not result in a code violation. As soon as you notice unethical behavior on the part of the supervisor, it would probably be a good time to start looking for a better supervisor.

CHALLENGE 4: It was summer and the majority of our agency's clients were scheduled for in-clinic sessions. A supervisor scheduled herself to supervise RBTs (including myself), but I never saw her once except when she said that she was going to bill for the session because she was "on site."

RBT RESPONSE: "So, you are going to bill for this session? You didn't actually supervise me, right?"

COMMENTARY: It's going to feel awkward to correct your BCBA and bring up something as serious as a billing problem, but as an RBT who is behaving ethically and is aware of their code of ethics, it's extremely important for you to ask questions like these. A great way to feel more confident in situations like these is to start your session telling your supervisor, "I am looking forward to reading your feedback." Prompt your supervisor for feedback so you aren't left in a situation where you or the supervisor is billing unethically.

What RBTs Need to Know About Billing for Insurance[1]

- Knowledge of CPT code guidelines for their services.
- Knowledge of in-session note requirements for their services; completing and signing immediately after session or same day of service.
- Appropriate application of this knowledge in each session.
- Timely submission of session notes and billing elements.
- Obtaining parent signatures according to company standards.
- Identify issues where this knowledge appears out of alignment and seek information from agency owner for gaps in knowledge or discussion of concerns.

More Details

In light of the incidents of fraud that were committed in South Florida in 2018, the significance of this Code items seems all the more relevant and important. In the South Florida situation, RBTs and people posing as RBTs were billing for ABA services for more hours than there were in a day! At one agency, this ranged from 26.5 to 67 billable hours per day across eight employees. At another agency, the company was billing for behavior analysis services even though the "therapists" were not qualified. This agency was required to refund more than $1 million to Medicaid. Other kinds of unethical conduct that fall under this Code include encouraging others to violate the law and passing misinformation on to colleagues that you know to be illegal or unethical.

1 This information is courtesy of Michele Silcox, CMRS, CEO/Co-Owner ABABilling.net.

Code 1.04 Test Yourself: Multiple-Choice Questions

1. As an RBT, you are working with a client in a clinic and can see that your BCBA plans to conduct supervision with you during your session. Your supervisor is at the clinic but never comes to observe you and is once again a no-show. You check your calendar and can see that your supervisor billed for that time. What now?
   a. You ask your supervisor if she had any feedback from the session. She replies, "No. Everything looked good." You assume she was just discreetly observing you and continue as usual.
   b. You don't really understand how billing works, so you just assume that everything was okay and this was all just a misunderstanding.
   c. Wait and see if it happens again; then you will know for sure that she is doing something unethical and can address it then.
   d. Let your supervisor know that you saw she was going to supervise you but never did. Tell the supervisor that you wanted to get more information about the supervision sessions. She informs you that what happened this time was a last-minute change and she plans to reschedule. You respond, "I noticed you had already billed for the session; is there something I am missing? It looks like a billing issue to me."
2. For an in-home session, as soon as you arrived at a client's home, the parent informed you that she would need to end the session an hour early. She also let you know that she waited to tell you until the day of the cancellation because she heard that you can still bill insurance for the entire time if you are given last-minute notice.
   a. You assume that the parent knows the insurance regulations better than you do, so you tell her, "Sounds good," and bill for the entire time.

b. You inform your supervisor of the situation, let her know you do not feel comfortable billing the entire time, and ask her to modify your session to end an hour earlier.
c. You text another coworker, who confirms that she has done this in the past, so you feel it is okay for you to do as well.
d. You feel uneasy about billing but really need the hours that week, so you bill the entire time.

3. One of the clients you work with receives services in both school sessions during the day and evening sessions after school. One day, you received a message from your supervisor that you needed to start transporting the client from school to home per the parent's request because having you transport the child fit better into the family's schedule. You were given no information on any specific goals to work on during the driving time but were instructed to bill for the entire session (including time spent driving). What should you do if this happens to you?
   a. It does not seem right, but you can assume the supervisor would not inform you to do anything unethical, so you do as you arc told.
   b. Start working on answering questions during the ride, as that is probably one of the client's current goals. Because you are running trials, you can feel comfortable that billing for that time.
   c. Inform your supervisor that it appears as if this change was made based on parental convenience rather than therapeutic purposes. Let the supervisor know you do not feel comfortable transporting the child or billing his insurance.
   d. You really need all the hours you can get, so go ahead and bill for the time (including driving). You could also choose to take the long way to the client's house.

For correct answers, see Appendix A

FOR FURTHER READING

Schmitz, S., & Silcox, M. (2019). *Revenue Cycle Management ABA Therapy*. Buzzards Bay, MA: Cape Cod Collaboration.

1.05 IF RBTs' ETHICAL RESPONSIBILITIES CONFLICT WITH EMPLOYER POLICIES, RBTs MUST BRING THE CONFLICT TO THEIR SUPERVISOR'S ATTENTION, DOCUMENT THAT THEY DID SO, AND DOCUMENT THE RESOLUTION

> *"It is important for RBTs . . . to have a good understanding of company policies before they accept a position with any organization."*

Quick Take

As an RBT, you should be using this Ethics Code as your guiding light when it comes to day-to-day decision-making within your company or organization. You might assume that your employer's policies are designed to protect client rights and safety and are in line with behavior analysis principles and values described in Code 1.01. Unfortunately, this may not always be true, so this Code reminds you to be sensitive to possible conflicts and prepared to try to resolve a disagreement if you encounter one in your work setting. If this happens, your first step is to talk to your BCBA supervisor and follow up with an email or memo so that your effort is documented (keep this in a safe place). Assuming there is a resolution, you will want to document this as well. If there is no resolution and you now feel uncomfortable with the tension this conflict is causing, you may need to reconsider your continued employment with this organization.

CHALLENGE 1: Phone dialogue between an RBT and her BCBA supervisor.

BCBA: "Hey, so Yami is going to be late today, but she won't be as late if you just pick her up on your way to work."

RBT: "Oh, but I thought it was against BACB policy for us to transport clients to or from the clinic?"

BCBA: "It technically is, but this is a favor to the family and I know you need the hours."

RBT RESPONSE: "I don't feel comfortable doing that. I read about this in the BACB Newsletter policy.[2] I'll just wait for her to arrive at the clinic and will bill according to the time she is here."

CHALLENGE 2: Your company highlights one client each month on their website by posting a picture and summary of the child's recent accomplishments. The parents love it and share these postings with the grandparents and friends. For a while, you thought this was a great way of showing the families how much you care. However, you recently found out this is unethical, as it exposes the client to the world, revealing that he most likely receives ASD, Developmental Disabilities (DD), or other behavioral services.

RBT TO OWNER: "I would like to show you something I recently found out." (opens Ethics book to Code 8.04 and RBT Ethics Code 2.05). "We should not be posting pictures of our clients on the website; they have a right to privacy and confidentially, and we are taking that away by exposing them. Look—it says it right here in the Code."

OWNER (not a BCBA): "Wow, that's news to me. We never meant any harm; we just wanted to celebrate how well our clients are doing. You are right: this is not okay, and I will make sure it stops and present a new policy to our board."

2 This is on page 2 of the April 2017 BACB Newsletter.

COMMENTARY: This was handled very professionally, and the owner was right to stop using testimonials and pictures; however, this ideal reaction may not always be the response you see, especially if the owner is not a BCBA. Having the owner change company policy on this would be a significant step forward to matching company policy with the RBT and BACB codes.

CHALLENGE 3: A client is extremely sick with a rising fever at 100°F and a rash that is spreading over his body, and his mother brought him to the clinic for therapy anyway. Typically, this child is constantly eloping, but today he is sitting in a chair with his head on his desk, sobbing. You called the mother and asked her to pick him up and said that he can't come back with a fever, even if the doctor says the rash is not contagious. It is against company policy to provide services to a client who has had a fever in the last 24 hours; however, your BCBA still scheduled home sessions for the following day and is expecting you to implement programs despite the client being so sick.

RBT TO MOM: "I don't feel comfortable implementing therapy with a client who is not physically healthy. He was constantly crying yesterday, and I could not get him to stop. He is not healthy enough for therapy. It is against company policy for us to be treating him since he had a fever within the last 24 hours. Therapy will not be effective, and we should not bill for that time."

COMMENTARY: To protect the other children, it is company policy for the child not to receive services within 24 hours of having a fever. It is the job of the BCBA to uphold company policy as well, but in this example, the BCBA was more worried about billing hours than the health of the client and the RBT. It is not a reasonable expectation for you to work with a sick client, nor would it be effective therapy if you did. This RBT was right to bring this to the attention of the BCBA.

CHALLENGE 4: When your client was running late for the session, you notified your supervisor. The supervisor responded, "Okay, just make sure you are preparing necessary stimuli for your session and reviewing programs and you can still bill for the entire time. It's company policy."

RBT RESPONSE: "Does the insurance company allow for you to bill like that? I thought that we could only bill for time spent actually spent conducting therapy."

BCBA: "It sure does; any time spent preparing or conducting therapy is included in the billing code."

RBT: "This makes me nervous; is there a way that I could look at that?"

COMMENTARY: There are a lot of different ways companies will try to get creative regarding billing codes, but those codes are there for a reason. As the RBT who will actually be submitting hours for your session, you need know what is allowed and what isn't. Your company should have a written policy for "late-parent" billing, and the RBT should not have to take responsibility for that decision. It is always best to bring any ethics questions regarding billing directly to your supervisor (in writing) to make sure you are covered in case of an audit.

"These company rules and regulations are typically found in a policy and procedure manual that you can ask to review before you sign on the dotted line."

More Details

It is important for RBTs as well as other behavioral staff to have a good understanding of company policies before they accept a position with any organization. These company rules and regulations are typically found in a *policy and procedure manual* that you can ask to review before you sign on the dotted line. This could be a daunting task since it might consist of a large binder, some of it written in legal language, with many subsections covering all aspects of the company's operation. You will be particularly interested in any section that has to do with RBT policies that might have to do with company dress code, your employment status, how you are paid, what happens if your client cancels a session, and so on. The other document you will want to read carefully is your contract with the organization; this will specify details of how you are supervised, warnings not to develop a dual relationship with the client, and possibly special clauses that prohibit revealing information about the company, known as a non-disclosure agreement. Some contracts also include a "non-compete" clause (more on this later) and a "notice of termination" clause where it specifies how much notice you need to give the company if you are going to quit.

Code 1.05 Test Yourself: Multiple-Choice Questions

1. Some co-workers invited you to go out for a burger after work. You were all wearing your company's shirt. It is against company policy to wear your shirt while out in the community and not on the clock. Your friends told you it was fine and that they wear the company-branded clothes in public all the time. How should you respond?
   a. "This sounds super fun, and if we all have our work shirts on, no one person can get in trouble."
   b. "I'm wearing my work shirt, so I'll eat quickly and leave right after I eat."
   c. "I will see you all at the restaurant. I am going to run home and change clothes."
   d. "Just no one take any pictures of me. We could be in trouble if these land on social media."

2. It is against company policy to take food from the clients' edibles cabinet, but you didn't bring any lunch and you got scheduled for another session. You've seen other therapists get food from the cabinet before and no one caught them. How should you respond?
   a. Stay out of the cabinet and have food delivered to the office.
   b. Quickly grab a bag of chips; something small from the cabinet is not a problem.
   c. Tell someone that you are getting food for a client.
   d. Eat fast and hope no one sees you.
3. Your supervisor, Dawn, asked you to stop by the office prior to going to your school and pick up a gift for one of the teachers for Teacher Appreciation Day. The supervisor asked you to give the gift to the teacher during your session. Dawn let you know that the company provides these gifts to all of the teachers as a way to show them "we care." What do you do?
   a. Your first step is to ask her what the gift is. If it is a small gift (school supplies, mug, etc.), you can give the gift to the teacher and not be in violation of any code items.
   b. Tell your supervisor that providing gifts to clients is against the Code and since the teacher is your client, you will not be able to give her the gift.
   c. Pick up the gift and give it to the teacher. This is a great way to pair yourself with a reinforcer and show the teacher you appreciate all that she does.
   d. Give the gift to the teacher, but make sure that you inform her it is from the company. Because you personally did not buy it, it is okay for you to give it to her.

For correct answers, see Appendix A

1.06 RBTs AVOID MULTIPLE RELATIONSHIPS WITH CLIENTS AND SUPERVISORS. IF THEY FIND THAT A MULTIPLE RELATIONSHIP HAS DEVELOPED DUE TO UNFORESEEN CIRCUMSTANCES, THEY INFORM THEIR SUPERVISOR AND WORK TO RESOLVE IT. IF THE MULTIPLE RELATIONSHIP INVOLVES THEIR SUPERVISOR, THE RBT SHOULD REPORT IT TO THE PERSON TO WHOM THEIR SUPERVISOR REPORTS

> *"You might be assigned to a client for in-home therapy as an RBT only to discover that one of the parents is your cousin or that you are neighbors with the family."*

Quick Take

A multiple relationship is one where you are involved with a client or supervisor as part of your job, and you are also involved in some other role with that same person. For example, you might be assigned to a client for in-home therapy as an RBT only to discover that one of the parents is your cousin or that you are neighbors with the family. In many cases, you may be assigned to work with a child whose parents want to treat you as if you were one of the family. These well-intentioned people want you to have dinner with them or go on family outings. They will often invite you to their child's birthday party. The primary concern is that in such a situation, you would very likely have your objectivity compromised. For example, an RBT who became friends with her client's parents might find it difficult to give them bad news regarding assessment results, a change of her therapy schedule, or a reduction in daily hours. Befriending clients or their families can create the impression of favoritism to others at your agency or clinic, and this can be damaging to your working relationship with other clients and supervisees.

Similar problems arise if a multiple relationship involves your supervisor. If your supervisor suggests that since you live in the same neighborhood, you could carpool to work, that close interaction twice daily would automatically create a multiple relationship between the supervisor and supervisee who have now become friends. If you were invited by your supervisor to attend a play where her child was performing, this would also create a dual relationship. If you felt you could not get out of this invitation and then found yourself invited to other activities with the supervisor ("Let's go to that yoga class together"), you might need to go to *her* supervisor to try to resolve this problem.

CHALLENGE 1: You are an RBT who is employed a few hours per week as a babysitter for a family whose child has recently been diagnosed with ASD. Your supervisor assigned you to the client's case, even though she knew you were still babysitting for the family.

RBT RESPONSE: I am going to tell my supervisor that I can't work with the client since I am also the babysitter. Even if I were to quit babysitting, the family would be expecting that same type of service from me. It would be unethical to provide anything other than ABA therapy.

COMMENTARY: This RBT was absolutely correct to discuss this issue with the BCBA and ask to be removed from the case. This would have easily been a multiple relationship; the family would have different expectations, and it would be unethical to work with this child.

CHALLENGE 2: A supervisor routinely entertains the RBTs from her work team at her home. She has invited some of them to her wedding. You just joined the team, and now she has approached you about meeting her at happy hour.

RBT RESPONSE: "I appreciate being included, but I am worried that it might look like a dual relationship."

COMMENTARY: This supervisor clearly creates dual relationships with supervisees, which is unethical for the

BCBA and for any RBT who accepts this invitation. It is important to be professional and have a good working relationship at the clinic, but meeting your supervisor for drinks after work is crossing the line.

CHALLENGE 3: A BCBA working at your company used to be a teacher at one of the local schools. The BCBA is related by marriage to the company owners. The school sends all of its student referrals solely to the company for which you are working, and they only consult with this BCBA.

RBT RESPONSE: You need to discuss this with the BCBA or the clinical director and explain how this is a multiple relationship and that it's violating Code 1.06. Your company should not be receiving all of the referrals, and other BCBAs should be hired to work with the clients in that school.

COMMENTARY: There are many different types of dual relationships, and it is important as an RBT to be aware of them. As the RBT, you need to be able to identify when a dual relationship is occurring and be able to discuss it with your supervisors if you are drawn into the dual relationship net.

CHALLENGE 4: Your supervisor sent you an email giving you information on a new client. The client name sounded familiar. When you arrived at the client's home and met the family, you realized that this is a family you knew from your old neighborhood. They reminded you that they became best friends with your parents after you left for college.

RBT RESPONSE: Thinking that this was going to be an easy assignment, you were eager to renew the acquaintance and start working with the child.

BCBA RESPONSE: After your first on-site supervision, your BCBA said, "You seemed awfully chummy with the family; what gives?" You explained the situation, and your supervisor said, "I'm pulling you off the case; this is clearly a dual relationship. I should document the fact that you thought this was okay, but since you are new here, I'm giving you just a verbal warning. You need to go study the RBT Ethics Code carefully."

COMMENTARY: The RBT was lucky that her supervisor caught this violation early before the relationship was more fully developed and that she received only a warning.

"Other examples of dual relationships include an RBT related to the owner who was hired by the owner's company, an RBT who was invited on vacations with the client's family, and a BCBA who developed a sexual relationship with an RBT who was a supervisee."

More Details

Dual relationships can create serious problems within a company and conflicts with other RBTs and supervisors, as well as problematic encounters with administrative staff. If an RBT becomes too friendly with a supervisor, it will soon be noticed by the other therapists. A friendship between the RBT and supervisor can result in favoritism shown to the RBT. Jealousy and animosity on the part of the other RBTs can easily arise and lead to rumors and allegations of even deeper, more controversial relationships. Some common morale problems involve complaints about the RBT receiving special privileges in the company, promotions, raises, more accommodating schedules, easier clients, and so on. Other examples of dual relationships include an RBT related to the owner who was hired by the owner's company, an RBT who was invited on vacations with the client's family, and a BCBA who developed a sexual relationship with an RBT who was a supervisee. Sadly, the list goes on and on and on. BCBAs need to be on the alert not to entrap RBTs into dual relationships such as inviting them for drinks after work, to their parties, or to birthday parties and weddings. As a final example, a BCBA and an RBT that the BCBA supervised had children about the same age who went to the same preschool. They would run into each other occasionally when picking up their children at school. This led to playdates, which led to running conversations at work that excluded other RBTs. This too-cozy relationship resulted in a complaint made to the clinical director about this obvious dual relationship and resulted in the RBT being transferred to another branch of the agency.

Remember to document any action that you take by putting your concerns in writing via email or a memo so that you will be covered if questions arise about your possible failure to let your supervisor or *her* supervisor know about a multiple relationship in your work environment.

Additional Multiple Relationships to Be Avoided

1. Business or professional relationships with client—A client proposes that you become a therapist or co-owner/investor at a private school they are creating.
2. Bartering for services—A family proposes that in exchange for you not charging them for billable hours that they will provide you with free meals at their restaurant.
3. Providing services to close friends, acquaintances, or family members—For example, a good friend has a child on the spectrum and they know that you are an experienced RBT. They ask if you would stop by their house and spend a little time with 2-year-old Andre and tell them if you think he would benefit from ABA therapy.

As another example, a parishioner from your church is out walking after Sunday services with her 4-year-old son, Skye. She introduces you to him, and you interact for a few minutes. Thirty minutes later, there is a message on your phone, and Skye's mom is asking, "What did you think of Skye? Do you think he needs therapy? Can you get him an appointment at your company?" You are not able to give an answer and say, "I'm sorry, this is not something I can do. I'm not qualified, and it would be against my Code of Ethics. But here is the number for the right person at my company; you can call and make an appointment."

4. Socializing with supervisors or clients—Your BCBA supervisor is getting married and invites you to the wedding. You need to thank him for the kind invitation but remind him that this would be a violation of Code 1.06.
5. Small-town contingencies—Small communities present special problems since there may be only one ABA company in town, everyone knows one another, and many are related by blood or marriage. Under such circumstances, you will have to work closely with your supervisor and clinical director to reduce whatever dual relationships you may have to the absolute minimum; otherwise, the entanglements can be all consuming.
6. Accepting gifts, asking for favors—In the *BACB Professional and Ethical Compliance Code for Behavior Analysts* Code 1.06 (d), it states, "Behavior analysts to do not accept *any* gifts," which we take to mean *zero*, and this would logically extend to asking a supervisor or client for a favor (see RBT Ethics Code 2.04 for reference). If you knew that your client's family ran an electronics business, it would be inappropriate to ask them if they could get you a good price on a new computer. Likewise, if they offer you a piece of the cake left over from Tami's fifth birthday party, you should decline. In both examples, dual relationships would be created by asking a favor or accepting the gift.

7. Giving gifts to clients or supervisors—It is customary in our culture for friends to give gifts to people on their birthday or on the occasion of special events in their lives such as graduation or a promotion. Note that we said this was common for "friends" to do, so if your client's parents are celebrating an anniversary, it would be inappropriate and actually unethical to give them a gift. The same would apply if your supervisor received an award or recognition. Other professions do not have a strict rule about giving or accepting gifts, so expect that there may be some strange looks coming your way when you say, "I'm sorry, this is not allowed by my RBT Ethics Code."

Code 1.06 Test Yourself: Multiple-Choice Questions

1. You are currently working at an agency and asked your BCBA for more hours. The clinical director overheard you and said that she could help you increase your income by paying you to babysit her children. How should you respond?
   a. "Perfect. I need the money and will be sure to keep my work issues separate."
   b. "That is nice of you to offer, but this would be a dual relationship and would be unethical."
   c. "How much do you pay per hour?"
   d. "Thank you for helping me."
2. One day, while in line at movie theater, you saw one of your school-based clients and his family. His mother introduced you to the uncle, whom you quickly recognized as an employee at a company your father owns. The uncle mentioned how you know each other and how he has heard such wonderful things about his family member's therapist. He cannot believe it is you. What do you do?

a. Contact your supervisor and inform her that you need to be taken off the case.
b. Let the uncle know that you cannot discuss anything regarding the client's case with him because you would then be in violation of the Code.
c. Just wait and see if it becomes a problem. You only interact with the uncle seldom, and most likely nothing will come up.
d. Nothing. The uncle and you do not have a direct relationship (only indirectly through your father), so you are not in violation of 1.06.

Code 1. 06 Test Yourself: True or False Questions

3. A dual relationship exists when an RBT is out partying with their supervising BCBA.
   True or False?
   True
   False
4. It is acceptable for the clinical director to hire someone as an RBT who used to be a hairdresser for the clinical director at the company. This is acceptable.
   True or False?
   True
   False

For correct answers, see Appendix A

1.07 RBTs DO NOT ENGAGE IN SEXUAL RELATIONSHIPS WITH CLIENTS OR SUPERVISORS. RBTs REFRAIN FROM SEXUAL RELATIONSHIPS WITH FORMER CLIENTS OR SUPERVISORS FOR AT LEAST TWO (2) YEARS FOLLOWING THE DATE THE WORKING RELATIONSHIP ENDED

> "A male RBT is providing services to child with a single mom; over time, they begin to engage socially."

Quick Take

A sexual relationship is a more intricate and complicated version of a dual relationship as discussed in 1.05. Situations like this are to be avoided at all costs: A male RBT is providing services to child with a single mom; over time, they begin to engage socially, perhaps after a therapy session or on a weekend. One thing leads to another, and the next thing you know, the RBT is spending the night at the client's home. The BCBA supervisor suspects that the RBT is more involved with the family than is proper and confronts the RBT, who denies everything. But then the mom drops a comment at a supervision session about how Rob, the RBT, is such a help at fixing things around the house. The BCBA asks point blank, "Are you seeing him?" to which she responds honestly, "Well, yes actually, we are dating, is that a problem? I don't want to get anyone in trouble." The BCBA advises the company of the situation, and the RBT is taken off this case and advised per Code 1.07 that he is not allowed to continue this relationship for a two-year cooling-off period. The RBT thinks about this for a few days and then turns in his resignation.

This Code also covers intimate relationships between RBTs and their supervisors, and the same rules apply. Anything beyond a working relationship is unacceptable and must be reported to the clinical director, and the appropriate changes of schedule or assignments must be made. If changes are not made, then both parties could be reported to the Board. If these two consenting adults wish to take their relationship to that next step, they must wait for a two-year period, and in the meantime, the supervisor cannot work with the RBT.

CHALLENGE 1: An RBT went to his supervisor and said, "I am developing feelings for Becky's mom, and I believe she feels the same. What do I do now?"

BCBA RESPONSE: "Thank you for alerting me to this, Alec. You could get in serious trouble if you let this go any further. I will be informing the mother I'm taking you off this case. You may not contact this mother again for another two years. There cannot be any contact between you and this client's mother."

COMMENTARY: The RBT did the right thing by bringing this to the attention of his supervisor. A situation like this can cause serious problems and needs to be addressed immediately.

CHALLENGE 2: You are an RBT who is supervised by a BCBA who has started scheduling you to work with your most preferred clients. The BCBA has also started scheduling you to get off earlier on Fridays. The supervisor began asking you what you do on weekends, and on Saturday night, the BCBA showed up at the club you mentioned you go to on Saturdays and wanted to know your plans for the following weekend. The BCBA supervisor has started giving you compliments and asked if you are dating anyone.

ADVICE TO RBT: You should not be discussing your private life with your supervisor. You are creating a dual relationship, and you are in violation of Code 1.07. This could evolve into a sexual relationship with your supervisor.

WHAT TO SAY: "I think it would be best if I transferred to a different supervisor, as I feel that our relationship has extended beyond supervisor-supervisee."

COMMENTARY: Regardless of sexual orientation or gender identity, it is unethical for RBTs to engage in any kind of relationship outside of work. Both you and your supervisor might be violating this code item, and you need to speak to the clinical director about working under another BCBA if this problem continues.

CHALLENGE 3: An RBT got a message from a family he used to work with after he left the company and moved to a nearby town. The family told him that the child was asking about him, and the parents would like to invite the RBT to stop by for a visit.

RBT RESPONSE: The RBT visits the client, and they continue to stay in touch.

COMMENTARY: Since this is a *former* client and just a social call, there is no problem. RBTs are allowed to maintain social relationships under these circumstances.

CHALLENGE 4: Jess is an RBT who works in the home with a client. The client's dad is usually home in the afternoon when Jess shows up to work with his daughter. Mr. Douglas is very friendly, observes the sessions carefully, and is obviously interested in learning about behavior analysis. After a number of weeks, Mr. Douglas told Jess to just call him "Doug" since that's what his friends call him. He has asked about Jess's interests and what she does on the weekends and mentioned how lonely he is since his wife works out of town so much. He implied that his wife may be having an affair. As a recent session was winding down, a babysitter showed up. Doug walked Jess out to her car and suggested she meet him at a local bar for drinks and appetizers.

RBT RESPONSE: "Sounds good; it's been a long week; why not."

COMMENTARY: This could go badly in so many ways both for parties. The dual relationship initiated by the father came on slowly and seemed natural to the RBT, but she should have stopped it at the point where he was walking her to her car and asking how she spends her non-work time. The RBT needs to meet with her supervisor immediately and ask to be removed from the case.

> *"In a recent case, an RBT doing her supervision hours for her master's degree was harassed and stalked by her BCBA."*

More Details

Sexual relationships that grow out of professional interactions with current clients can tarnish or destroy the reputation of all the parties, do damage to our profession, and cause serious emotional harm to the child client. This sort of intimate connection can begin innocently enough if the RBT engages in self-disclosure with the client, who is often the parent. This opens the door to conversations where the client feels it is acceptable to have a dialogue about personal issues, and this can slowly lead to sexual misconduct. The RBT can easily lose professional objectivity and develop a loyalty toward the client that competes with their required objectives for the child client. In such situations, RBTs may keep certain information about the parent from the BCBA supervisor or modify, without approval, the behavior plan to make it easier for the parent to implement. This, of course, results in the child client showing less progress. If the child observes intimate behavior on the part of the RBT toward the parent, this is likely to cause confusion and force an emotional wedge between the child and the parents.

Recent history has shown that when a power dynamic exists in a work setting that exploitation by the more powerful person can easily happen. Examples of producers preying on young female actresses, sports stars victimizing spouses, and corporate executives taking advantage of junior employees are all in the news. Less known are the cases of BCBAs exploiting their position with supervisees and young RBTs, but the result can be the same if the RBT feels powerless and unable to get out of the situation for fear of being fired. In a recent case, an RBT who was completing her supervision hours for her master's degree was harassed and stalked by the BCBA who controlled her work schedule and hours worked. Since this person was also the owner of the company where the RBT/student was placed, the RBT felt there was no one who would listen to her appeal. Eventually, she did speak with the BCBA's wife, and a messy divorce ensued.

Code 1.07 Test Yourself: Multiple-Choice Questions

1. Your supervising BCBA seems to spend a lot of time with a certain RBT. This RBT and BCBA have been seen outside of working getting coffee together or getting dinner. You also start to notice that this RBT has been choosing which cases she wants to work on and misses work frequently without any penalties. How should you respond?
   a. Keep your head down and ignore what is going on. It's none of your business.
   b. Cover the RBT's sessions because you believe in love.
   c. Record what you have observed and get some evidence of the differential treatment. Take this to the clinical director because the BCBA and the RBT are violating Code 1.07.
   d. Post this story on social media, and others will handle the situation for you.

Test Yourself: True or False Questions

2. After leaving your job at a particular agency, you saw your former BCBA supervisor at a coffee shop. During a really pleasant conversation, you realized how much you have in common with your former supervisor. It is okay if you start dating this person.
   True or False?
   True
   False
3. You are an RBT and you and your current BCBA supervisor have always gotten along. You clearly have a lot in common with your supervisor. Asking him out on a date is permitted.
   True or False?
   True
   False

For correct answers, go to Appendix A

1.08 RBTs RECOGNIZE THAT THEIR PERSONAL PROBLEMS AND CONFLICTS WITH OTHERS MAY IMPACT THEIR ABILITY TO PERFORM THEIR DUTIES AND REFRAIN FROM PROVIDING SERVICES WHEN THIS IS THE CASE

Quick Take

> "If you in any way feel that you might not be fulfilling your obligations to your clients or your workplace, it is time to have a heart-to-heart talk with your supervisor."

It could happen that you develop a problem or two in your personal life. Some people develop chronic illnesses, experience messy breakups with long-time partners, or become addicted to substances. If you experience any of these problems, as in the case of any practitioner, your obligation is to make sure that personal issues or conflicts do not interfere with your ability to deliver quality services to your clients. Assuming that you have a good working relationship, this is probably best handled by talking with your supervisor. If you in any way feel that you might not be fulfilling your obligations to your clients or your workplace, a heart-to-heart talk with your supervisor can help you sort out your options. Some of those may involve taking a leave of absence for a period of time while you get your life in order. During this time, you need to make sure that your supervisor has made arrangements to cover your clients.

CHALLENGE 1: While in a graduate program for ABA, you are working as an RBT and pursuing certification. As you get further along in your first semester, you notice your workload quickly building up. At first you were able to stay afloat, but now you find yourself turning in assignments late, forgetting to read pertinent emails on protocol changes, updating your client's program infrequently, arriving late to sessions from sleeping in, and consuming too much Red Bull. You know you are not putting in the quality of work you should be in school or work, and you feel so behind, you're not sure of how to catch up.

RBT TO BCBA: "I'm feeling overwhelmed and concerned that I am starting to fall behind on my work. I need some help; is there anything that you can do?"

BCBA TO RBT: "Thank you for bringing this to my attention. I know how difficult it can be while you are in graduate school. I have some RBTs who would be happy to take some of this busywork off of your hands so that you can have more time to focus on your other responsibilities. Let's start with that and plan a meeting in a week to regroup."

COMMENTARY: Admitting that you need help can be a difficult task, but it is your responsibility to ensure you are taking on only as much as you can handle. A good supervisor will understand and provide you with the proper support to help you get back on track. In the event that your supervisor does not respond so well, you should be prepared with a back-up plan to ensure you do not fall further behind.

CHALLENGE 2: The migraines you had your senior year of high school appear to have resurfaced. Back then, it was because you were head cheerleader, played flute in the orchestra, were quite active in honor society, and were class president in addition to working part time at a sporting goods store. Your physician put you on some medication, prescribed massage therapy, and advised you to drop two of these and quit the job. You followed her advice and felt better in a few weeks (although you missed the flute, cheering, and income). Now you have a full RBT caseload and you are taking two night courses at community college.

WHAT TO DO: Migraines are serious and can lead to other medical complications. What worked for you previously might work again, so schedule an appointment with your physician. This time, you also need to speak to your BCBA supervisor to see if you can get a reduction in your caseload. If you start missing work or making mistakes on your data collection or graphing, you could get fired. Follow the advice in the COMMENTARY for Challenge 1, and you should get through this crisis.

CHALLENGE 3: You are experiencing a messy break-up and regularly receive texts from your ex threatening to go to your place of work and inform the company owner of sensitive information you brought up when venting about work-related frustrations. (He was a good listener; you have to give him that.)

RBT RESPONSE: You decide that your ex-boyfriend is just being emotional and text him back in the middle of a client session, "I'd like to see you try."

COMMENTARY: This challenge is clearly unethical, and the RBT's personal life is interfering with the ability to implement treatments effectively. The better response would be to meet ASAP with your supervisor. Although you are uncertain if the ex will actually act on these threats, this potential interaction is something your owner should be aware of so that she can prepare accordingly. As uncomfortable as it may be, you would rather be safe than sorry. Note that discussing confidential client information with your ex was a violation of Code 2.08. You also need to own up to this with your supervisor.

CHALLENGE 4: Roger, your first-year dorm roommate, got you interested in gambling on college sports. Roger had developed a "system" for picking winners that seemed foolproof, and he made enough money to fly to Las Vegas once a month. Then he dropped out of school, and you haven't heard from him since. What was once a fun hobby, just a minor distraction from boring course work, has become an addiction that is beginning to take its toll—your steady girlfriend of two years has left you, depression is starting to set in, you are anxious, you've maxed out your credit card, and your bookie is calling you at all hours.

RBT RESPONSE: You ask for a raise and more hours at the company where you are a tech.

BCBA SUPERVISOR: "Brandon, I've been meaning to talk to you about your work here at ABC Health. I'm not happy with how things are going with your cases, the client doesn't feel you are focused, your reports are full of errors and omissions, and it looks like you might be inflating your hours. There will be no more hours, and no raise. Instead, I want you to meet with Lori in HR. I'm not allowed to ask what the problem is, but I'm sure they can set up some counseling for you."

> *"The natural tendency when you realize that your life is falling apart is to try to cover it up so that you don't get fired from your job."*

More Details

The natural tendency when you realize that your life is falling apart is to try to cover it up so that you don't get fired from your job. An ex-boyfriend that is stalking you, an alcohol problem that is producing hangovers that last past noon, or even a credit-card problem can be distracting, worrisome, and disturbing. Any of these or similar problems can make you late to the clinic or the home of a client. Showing up drunk or hung over is totally unacceptable, so you may call in sick or make up an excuse, "My car won't start, Mrs. Hall, so I am going to miss my session with Elijah this afternoon. I am so sorry. Can we make this up on the weekend?" Excuses and lies will catch up with you quickly, so the best solution is to seek help immediately and talk with your supervisor or the HR department if your company has one. Some companies will arrange a leave of absence that can be used to get your life back together, so by all means, take advantage of these services.

Code 1.08 Test Yourself: Multiple-Choice Questions

1. Having argued with your boyfriend all night, you are driving to work with a killer headache, and you are exhausted from the fight. As you begin a session, the client starts to engage in an emotional outburst, and you start to cry as well. How should you respond?
   a. Keep crying together because you are both sad. This will make you feel better.
   b. Leave the session and go home after telling another therapist you are leaving.
   c. Find your supervisor, and explain that you should have called in sick today. Finish the session, but ask for the rest of the day off.
   d. Tell at the client to stop crying because she doesn't have real problems.

Code 1.08 Test Yourself: True or False Question

2. As soon as you leave work, you head to your favorite dive bar for a few cool ones. This doesn't mean anything; it's not really a serious problem, although you have had to call in "sick" once or twice a week with a serious hangover. This is not a violation of Code 1.08.
   True or False?
   True
   False

For correct answers, go to Appendix A

1.09 RBTs FOLLOW THROUGH ON OBLIGATIONS AND CONTRACTUAL COMMITMENTS WITH HIGH-QUALITY WORK, AND THEY DO NOT MAKE COMMITMENTS THEY CANNOT KEEP

> "A contract is a commitment, in writing, with teeth, so read it carefully."

Quick Take

Becoming a Registered Behavior Technician could be your first job with important responsibilities that can affect another person, most likely a child, in a meaningful way. Since you will be spending so many hours per week with your client conducting language and social skills training as well as possibly implementing behavior-reduction programs, it is very likely that you signed a contract with your company. This contract is a legally binding agreement that outlines your job duties and states the number of hours you will work each month, what your rate of pay will be, the length of the commitment if they are paying for your training, the company dress code, grounds for termination, and possibly other details that will govern your work life for the next year or two. Signing a contract should be taken very seriously, since violating such an agreement could result in your being sued or taken to court where you may have to pay a damages award. A contract is a commitment, in writing, with teeth, so read it carefully and consider having someone else look it over, too, especially if you know someone who runs a business or is possibly an attorney.

CHALLENGE 1: As a Lead RBT, your responsibilities include such tasks as creating materials, updating programs, and sending team update emails. You want to complete these responsibilities, but your supervisor often fails to schedule you time to work on them, and when she does, it is spontaneous and inconsistent. You try to make it work in the time you have but can see that you are not meeting your responsibilities.

WHAT NOT TO DO: You decide that since the supervisor isn't scheduling time for these duties, you aren't going to complete the work that is required. Your attitude is if she wants it done, then she needs to put it on your schedule.

WHAT *TO* DO: Go to your supervisor and be somewhat assertive in asking for the training and supervision you need.

COMMENTARY: This RBT had been promoted to Lead Tech, and with that come more responsibilities and the training necessary to meet these new requirements.

CHALLENGE 2: To ensure programs can be updated as necessary, the BCBA who supervises you has consistently reiterated the importance of entering the client's data before you leave the clinic for the day. Near the end of one session, you begin talking to one of your coworkers, who suggests you go out for pizza.

WHAT NOT TO DO: You both decide to leave early and plan to enter the data later. This should not be a big deal, as the BCBA has already left for the day and probably won't notice.

WHAT *TO* DO: Stay and finish your data as instructed prior to leaving the clinic. Your BCBA wouldn't ask you to do this unless it was important, and, knowing that insufficient data may result in detrimental effects on your client, your social life can wait.

COMMENTARY: Code 1.09 illustrates the importance of following through with obligations. When you commit to a request your BCBA made, it is your responsibility make sure the work gets completed.

CHALLENGE 3: With three years' experience, you are an RBT who is pursuing your AA degree in social sciences. You believe that you are entitled to more responsibilities at work because despite multiple on-site observation sessions, various forms of feedback, and even treatment integrity checklists by your BCBA, you are not still performing at a professional level implementing programs with clients. You are willing to learn and believe that your lack of progress is not a motivation problem.

WHAT NOT TO DO: You frequently complain to the other RBTs and even the receptionist about how the agency is treating you unfairly.

WHAT *TO* DO: Schedule a meeting with your BCBA to ask for more responsibilities and the opportunity to learn more about the actual work that a BCBA does. You tell your BCBA that you are available for additional training any time. Your BCBA starts asking you to make stimuli for clients, enter data, and start training newly hired therapists. Your BCBA asked you to have the stimuli made by the next session, but you did not get it finished.

WHAT *NOT* TO DO: Hope that, since your BCBA is also extremely busy, it won't be noticed that you didn't get all of the work done.

CHALLENGE 4: You have been an RBT for nearly two years, but you aren't sure if you would like to pursue further credentials. You ask your BCBA for more responsibilities and the opportunity to learn more about the actual work that a BCBA does. You also say that you are available for any time the BCBA has to teach you. As a result, she asks you to make stimuli for clients, enter data, and start training newly hired therapists. Your BCBA specifically asks you to have the stimuli made by the next session, but you did not get this task finished.

WHAT NOT TO DO: You assume your BCBA is also extremely busy and probably won't notice that you didn't get all of the work done.

WHAT *TO* DO: If you are asking for more responsibility, then you need to step up your game and make sure that you absolutely follow through with every commitment you make, no matter how small.

COMMENTARY: Being labeled a *slacker* at work is now not only an ethics code violation but just not as cool as it was in high school.

"A child's life is at stake here, and you are the person who makes a difference every single day. This is why this Code item mentions the importance of keeping your commitment to the client and the company."

More Details

The nature of RBT work is that you become quite close to the child client and the family. Your work very quickly becomes an *obligation* more than a job. What you do is a commitment to a person who needs your help, desperately, with a palpable payoff. As an RBT, you can actually see improvements in the client's behavior in real time and enjoy the natural consequences of your hard work. If you have signed a contract that says that you will stay with the company, this is your commitment, but your obligation to the client is even more important. This work is not like a summer job selling hotdogs at the local ball field or making ice cream cones down at the neighborhood ice cream shoppe. A child's life is at stake here, and you are the person who makes a difference every single day. This is why this Code item mentions the importance of keeping your commitment to the client and the company. Unexpected life circumstances might force you to resign from your job, but out of your obligation to the client, the ethical thing to do is give plenty of notice. When resigning, 30 days notice is considered appropriate. You should work closely with your supervisor to transition your cases to the next RBT who will take over the behavior plans in a seamless fashion.

Code 1.09 Test Yourself: Multiple-Choice Questions

1. You are an RBT who is moving in two months to a new city where you found work at a behavioral clinic. You have not told your current company yet. How should you respond?
   a. Wait until the last two weeks and put in your notice.
   b. Give a 30-day notice that you will be leaving.
   c. Wait until the last week because you are only an RBT and don't really have any paperwork or anything to take care of.
   d. Don't tell your current company and just stop showing up.
2. You have been coming to your company's research meetings for a few weeks, and it's your turn to present an article. You signed up three weeks prior to bring an article but forgot. The other members stressed that in order to participate, you must follow through with your commitments. How should you respond?
   a. Just move on and ignore any further mention of the issue.
   b. Stop coming to the meetings.
   c. Apologize, and say that you were wrong, you know it's part of the code to uphold obligations, and you will do better in the future.
   d. Never sign up for anything in the future.
3. You signed a contract in your role of a Lead RBT that states you are responsible for two hours of treatment planning for your client every week. However, each week, you find yourself really only needing an hour or less to complete of your updates. How should you respond?
   a. Bill for the entire two hours regardless of the time spent working. You are still completing the necessary amount of work but are just quicker than others.
   b. Use the extra time to work on responding to other work-related emails and continue to bill the full amount.

c. Take your time when completing the treatment planning to drag it out to match the amount of time provided.
d. Talk with your supervisor on what other treatment planning can be completed when you have additional time, or look into modifying the allotted amount of time.

Code 1.09 Test Yourself: True or False Question

4. Planning on obtaining your RBT credential, you interviewed at a company where you can receive your supervision hours. Congratulations! You were hired. The company presented you with a contract that specified that you will agree to stay on for one year once you earn your RBT because the company will be paying for your RBT training and test. You signed the contract. Six months later, you earned your RBT but now want to leave to go to another company that pays more per hour. It is unethical to break this contract.

   True or False?
   True
   False

For correct answers, go to Appendix A

1.10 RBTs DO NOT MAKE FALSE, DECEPTIVE, MISLEADING, EXAGGERATED, OR FRAUDULENT PUBLIC STATEMENTS ABOUT THEIR WORK OR QUALIFICATIONS

Quick Take

Misleading a company during a job interview about your familiarity with certain kinds of cases could result in your being assigned to clients that you are

> "Some RBTs are captivated with social media and may be tempted to brag on the internet about their prowess as a therapist."

not prepared to handle. If you suggest that you are experienced with aggressive or self-injurious teens and are assigned to work with such clients but have no idea what you are doing, both you and the clients could get seriously injured. Or, if in talking to the parents you imply that they are free to discuss their personal problems, you may find yourself caught up in a deep-rooted family dispute that could get you fired. Some RBTs are captivated with social media and may be tempted to brag about their prowess as a therapist on the internet or discuss a famous client. RBTs should be aware that this information could easily get back to their employer, who would not take kindly to this exposure of their clients.

CHALLENGE 1: Madison, an RBT, has been working in the field of ABA for a few months. Madison is excited about all of the progress he sees on the job. He is working with an ASD client who is close to phasing out of services entirely. He feels strongly that ABA "cured" his autism and has begun posting on social media about ABA and its ability to completely eradicate ASD symptoms.

RBT RESPONSE: Another RBT saw these posts and immediately sent Madison the following message: "These posts need to be removed. Although ABA has been effective in treating various behaviors associated with ASD, there is no empirical evidence to support that it is a 'cure' for ASD. I fully understand your excitement about ABA, but we need to make sure we are not issuing deceptive statements regarding its effectiveness and misleading families to believe it will cure their child."

COMMENTARY: The second RBT is correct that Madison made false and exaggerated statements that could easily confuse the public and create false hopes for parents. This is clearly a violation of Code 1.10 (the second RBT also did the right thing by reaching out to Madison and resolving this informally per Code 1.13).

CHALLENGE 2: At a state conference, an RBT was introduced by the chair of a panel in front as a BCBA expert on feeding disorders. (This was factually incorrect; the RBT had only taken two graduate courses toward her master's degree and had only worked as an assistant under a faculty member.) There were more than 200 people in the audience.

RBT RESPONSE: The RBT did not correct the chair but gave her presentation and answered a few questions at the end.

COMMENTARY: The RBT was in violation of Code 1.10 in that she allowed a false statement to be made in public about her qualifications, thus leading audience members to perhaps give more weight to her comments. Someone in the audience should have approached her afterward and given her feedback on this omission.

CHALLENGE 3: An RBT who recently joined a new company has been heard multiple times talking about how much she loves to work with problem behaviors. She told her new supervisor that at her previous clinic, "I only worked with clients with severe problem behaviors; do you want to see my scars?" The RBT is being trained on a new client who has moderate SIB (no tissue damage) and a few documented elopement attempts. At recess, the client raced across the playground, jumped a short fence, and made it across two lanes of traffic to a 7–11 store. The RBT received standard introductory behavior training, but the supervisor decided to allow the RBT to work independently on the case due to all of her previous experience. The first day the RBT was on her own, the client engaged in a new behavior, aggression. The therapist got hurt and asked to go home. When the BCBA asked the next day what happened, the RBT told the BCBA that she did not get adequate training and is uncomfortable with problem behavior.

RBT RESPONSE: This RBT has violated code 1.10 multiple times. She told her new supervisor that she had experience with problem behavior, prefers clients who engage in problem behaviors, and was ready to handle a case on her own. She was dishonest about her previous experience and is blaming her minor injury on her trainer.

COMMENTARY: This RBT is putting herself and the client at risk by lying about her work experience. As the RBT, you are there to help and teach the client, and if you aren't knowledgeable about their specific behavioral issues, you are endangering the client and others.

CHALLENGE 4: A newly credentialed RBT was interviewing at a clinic that serves families whose first language is Spanish. The company was looking to hire more RBTs, but they needed to be able to speak Spanish. The RBT took one Spanish class in high school, and was not proficient by any means. During the interview, the clinical director asked the RBT if she was fluent in Spanish.

RBT RESPONSE: "I have taken Spanish classes and studied one summer in Chile after my junior year of high school. I feel comfortable speaking Spanish and would be able to work with these families and properly translate all of the ABA terms for them."

COMMENTARY: After the interview, this company did a spot check of this applicant's resume and discovered she has never left the country, let alone done a summer study abroad in Chile. The RBT violated code 1.10. She not only misrepresented her experience with Spanish but also exaggerated her ability to translate technical ABA terminology into another language just to get the job.

"Misleading others about your skills or previous experience represents not only poor judgment on your part but also leads to a lack of trust."

More Details

False statements in the public arena are a serious ethical violation of Code 1.03 (*RBTs are truthful and honest*), and they are in violation of employer policies against breaking confidentiality. This means that doing so is a fireable offense. Misleading others about your skills or previous experience represents not only poor judgment on your part but also leads to a lack of trust. If you would lie about your proficiency as an RBT, what else would you fabricate? And does this mean that you might also have a tendency to reveal confidential information about clients or the company the company for which you work?

Code 1.10 Test Yourself: Multiple-Choice Question

1. The clinical director of a clinic that specializes in treating feeding disorders in children with autism is looking to hire RBTs that have experience in this area. Despite the fact that Ursula has never worked on a single feeding problem case, she decided to interview for a position at the clinic. The clinical director asked Ursula if she had any experience with feeding problems. How should she respond?
   a. I absolutely do. The majority of the cases I worked on at my last clinic involved feeding programs.
   b. No, I do not have any experience, but I am looking to gain experience in this area. I would really like to learn more about the different problem behaviors that can be treated with ABA.
   c. No, I don't have experience but I am a hard worker and I was hoping you would still give me the job.
   d. I think that behavior programs are similar enough that I could do this job.

Code 1.10 Test Yourself: True or False Question

2. Having failed the RBT exam three times, you are a behavior therapist who doesn't want to give up. You have moved

to a new city and are interviewing at a new clinic that only hires those who have their RBT. You wrote that you do have your RBT on your resume. This is okay since you are certain you will pass this time.

True or False?

True

False

For correct answers, go to Appendix A

1.11 RBTs PROVIDE A CURRENT AND ACCURATE SET OF CREDENTIALS (E.G., DEGREES, CERTIFICATIONS) TO CLIENTS, EMPLOYERS, AND SUPERVISORS UPON REQUEST. CHANGES TO CERTIFICATION STATUS MUST BE IMMEDIATELY REPORTED TO EMPLOYERS AND SUPERVISORS

> "When interviewing you for a job, your employer wants to know what your capability is and where you might fit into the organization."

Quick Take

Your credentials represent your background in ABA, your professional experience, and any specialty training that you might have had along the way. When interviewing you for a job, your employer wants to know what your capability is and where you might fit into the organization. Are you just a "newbie" RBT that will require a lot of supervision or a seasoned behavior tech that might be perfect for a Lead RBT slot that has just come open? If you are in a graduate program and looking for supervision hours, your employer will want to know how many hours you need to accrue. Your diplomas and certificates will let them know where you stand and how much time they will need to invest in you. If you are hired, your supervisor will be eager to learn about your background and experience working with previous clients, so any documentation you can provide will assist with the process of assigning you to client cases. Copies of previous behavior plans you have implemented (with names and other identifying information redacted, of course), functional analyses you have conducted, or reports that you have prepared are also forms of credentials that are useful. Finally, although it is not likely, the clients you work with may ask for some documentation that proves you are who you say you are, so it would be good to have information on where you got your RBT training. Clients might appreciate being able to verify your information by being provided with the link to the BACB.com website.

CHALLENGE 1: To expand your skills beyond your basic RBT credential, you were previously trained and certified at the *Practitioner 1* level in Professional Crisis Management (PCM). However, you've been busy with your upcoming wedding plans and somehow allowed your certification to lapse. One day, you received an urgent call from your supervisor to help transport a client to a safe room.

WHAT NOT TO SAY: "Sure, I'm on my way."

WHAT *TO* SAY: "I'm so sorry, I forgot to re-up my PCM certification; I will go find someone that can help."

COMMENTARY: The RBT violated Code 1.11 by not informing the company of a change of status, that is, failure to re-up the PCM training. Your next highest priority at this point is to contact the PCM instructor at your company, schedule the training, and renew your certification.

CHALLENGE 2: You just began working at a company and recently took your RBT exam but did not pass. Even though you have not passed, your company allows you to work with private-pay clients. You are training with a new client, and the Lead RBT introduces you to the client's mother by saying, "I'd like you to meet Ashton, our newest RBT."

RBT RESPONSE: "I actually have not obtained my RBT credential yet, but I have all my hours, so I will just need to pass my exam. It is so nice to meet you, and I look forward to working with you."

COMMENTARY: Although it may be an uncomfortable correction to make on the spot, Ashton must ensure that she is accurately representing herself in the field of ABA. Leading a client to believe she has a credential that she does not is unethical and certainly in violation of 1.11.

CHALLENGE 3: Although you have not taken the RBT exam yet, you are scheduled to take the test in a few weeks. You've decided to interview with an agency and get a job in place while you wait to take the test. The agency where you are interviewing only hires therapists who have completed their RBT training and passed the test. You wrote on your resume that you are an RBT, and during the interview, the clinical director asked you when you earned your RBT credential.

RBT RESPONSE: You tell them that you just received the credential a few weeks ago and you feel comfortable working with many different types of clients and are looking forward to learning about new clients.

COMMENTARY: You are not an RBT yet, and you should not be advertising yourself as an RBT. You have not taken the exam, which means you are not an RBT and should not be interviewing for an RBT position. You should have told the clinical director that you plan on taking the exam in a few weeks, and if you pass the exam, you could contact them then.

> *"Individuals with no background in child development or therapy were taking a 40-hour RBT crash course in one weekend."*

More Details

There was a period in Florida (circa 2015) where the word got around that there was an abundance of jobs in human services, that entry to this rapidly growing field was easy, and that take-home pay was generous. Individuals with no background in child development or therapy were taking a 40-hour RBT *crash course* in one weekend. Despite having this training, they did not bother to take the RBT Competency Assessment, or they took it and did not pass. These individuals represented themselves as legitimate RBTs to their new employers, eventually got caught, and were charged with fraud. Several companies were charged with insurance fraud as well. If the employers had required applicants to produce their RBT credentials, none of this would have happened.

Code 1.11 Test Yourself: Multiple-Choice Questions

1. You have been an RBT for two years now, and you are preparing for your BCaBA exam. You have taken the necessary courses and have all of the supervision hours necessary, but you can't sit for the BCaBA for a few months. Your RBT renewal is due in the next few weeks. You don't see the point in paying for the RBT renewal since you have to pay for the BCaBA exam, so you decide to not renew your RBT. Your supervisor asks if you submitted your renewal.
   a. "Oh no, I forgot to do that. I will submit it immediately."
   b. "Actually, I decided to not renew it since I am going to sit for the BCaBA, and I don't have the money to pay for both."
   c. "Oh yeah. I turned it in, and it was accepted. So, I am fine to keep working as an RBT."
   d. "When do I have to renew that?"
2. As soon as you applied for a role as a Lead RBT, your employer asked you to send redacted copies of previous

behavior plans, assessments, and protocol write-ups so they can get an idea of your writing experience. All of your previous work has been written with the assistance of your BCBA, and although you wrote many portions of it, she completed much of it and heavily rewrote the parts you did write. What should you do?

a. Turn it in. You worked on it, so turning it in as your own work would not be a lie and is not in violation.
b. Tell your prospective employer that you have no experience in job-related writing. Everything that you did complete was reviewed and edited by your BCBA, so it would be unethical to claim you have written anything.
c. Provide your pre-edited drafts and explain how you previously worked with your supervisor in write-up development.
d. Only give the portions that you assisted in writing. Even though they were edited, they were initially your writing, so you are being truthful in providing your work.

Code 1.11 Test Yourself: True or False Question

3. A new company that treats eating disorders is interviewing for RBTs, and you have decided to interview. On your résumé, it says that you attended a week-long workshop that resulted in a certificate of completion. You provide the certificate, and the clinical director asks you a few questions pertaining to the workshop and your experience working with feeding problems. You really did attend a workshop, but the workshop was actually one day long. This is just a minor error and nothing to worry about.

   True or False?
   True
   False

For correct answers, go to Appendix A

1.12 RBTs OBTAIN PERMISSION TO USE TRADEMARKED OR COPYRIGHTED MATERIALS AS REQUIRED BY LAW. RBTs PROVIDE CITATIONS THAT RECOGNIZE THE INTELLECTUAL PROPERTY OF OTHERS, INCLUDING TRADEMARK AND COPYRIGHT SYMBOLS

Quick Take

> "Violating copyright and trademarks can result in criminal charges and is clearly unethical."

You might decide to use a certain motto that is popular in the culture or a logo that you particularly like on a t-shirt that you propose to sell online for a worthy cause or to make some quick cash. You need to know that these symbols and expressions are intellectual property and that they have owners who could sue you if you do not have permission to use them on a shirt. A trademark ™ symbol or ® (registered trademark) appears somewhere on the image or expression and is the legal way of informing you that you cannot just copy and paste the marks on something you produce. This might be a special symbol such as the golden arches for McDonalds™ or an expression, such as Star Wars™ by Lucasfilms. These are forms of intellectual property owned by a person or a business. You are likely to see the copyright © symbol on printed materials such as books and training materials. This means that you need permission to make copies (that's right, on a copy machine) of this material. The most frequent violation is by an agency that uses certain tests routinely with clients, and rather than contacting the copyright owner and asking permission, they act like pirates and make copies when they need them. Violating copyright and trademarks can result in criminal charges, damages, or payment of legal fees, and this is clearly unethical.

CHALLENGE 1: You are working at a clinic that utilizes the Verbal Behavior-Milestones Assessment and Placement

Programs (VB-MAPP), and your supervisor informs you she will be training you on how to use it. Your supervisor then hands you a blank book and asks you to make copies of the assessment for your client.

RBT RESPONSE: You go to the mailroom and, with the help of the assistant, carefully make the required duplicates. You are motivated to learn more about how programs are created and how the VB-MAPP is administered.

COMMENTARY: It is unethical to reproduce the VB-MAPP Protocol or Guide since they are copyrighted. The clinic where you work should be purchasing a license for each learner (there are discounts for bulk orders). Most of the training materials in ABA are generated by professionals working with publishers who produce and distribute their work, and these works are copyrighted. Look for the © symbol in the front of the book, which means that you need to seek written permission from the publisher to duplicate the materials. There are legal penalties for copyright infringement that can range from $200 to $150,000 plus attorney fees and court costs.

CHALLENGE 2: Another RBT is showing you how to make Picture Exchange Communication System (PECS) picture icons that she downloaded from the web. She says that you can just copy the images to your laptop and print them whenever you need to make the cards.

RBT RESPONSE: "I checked these out on the web. It says, 'The purchaser is granted permission to download and print this item for noncommercial individual or single classroom use only. This file and finished product are copyright protected and is not to be shared or resold.' I don't feel comfortable doing this; the company should purchase these materials; copying could be illegal."

COMMENTARY: It may seem harmless, but this type of copying still violates Code 1.12. The company should purchase these picture icons and follow the copyright law.

CHALLENGE 3: Wanting to do everything you can to promote the work you do, you sign up for an autism awareness walk and help with fundraising. You think that more people need to know about the BACB and how to become an RBT, so you have a shirt made that prominently features the BACB logo. There is a BCBA at the walk who notices your shirt and says, "So, did you write to the BACB and get permission to copy and reprint their logo?"

RBT RESPONSE: "Well, no, but I'm sure the BACB would love to be a part of this event."

COMMENTARY: The BACB logo is trademarked, and you cannot use the logo without the permission of the BACB. They will most likely not want their logo on your shirt, even though they support any effort to raise awareness for behavior analysis treatment.

"It is in our culture's best interest to protect these creative people and their works from those who would steal or pirate them for their own benefit."

More Details

To understand copyright and trademark protection, we have to start with the concept of intellectual property (IP). Artists, writers, poets, playwrights, designers, and other creative, innovative people work hard to come up with new ideas that are in the public interest. IP rights assure them that they will receive some financial benefit or at least recognition from what they have invented or created; it is unethical (and basically stealing) to take this from them. If IP rights are not protected, then the primary incentive to be creative is removed, and our world will be the lesser for it. It is in our culture's best interest to protect creative people and their works from those who would steal or pirate them for their own benefit.

Code 1.12 Test Yourself: Multiple-Choice Question

1. Close to graduating with your bachelor's degree, you discovered that your university was hosting a job fair soon, and you wanted your agency represented. Someone told you to start making brochures with your agency's logo and the BACB logo for handouts at a booth. When your clinical director found out what you were doing, he told you that you can't use these logos without permission. He also said, "As an RBT, you don't have the authority to develop marketing materials for the company or commit us to have a booth without my permission." How should you respond?
   a. "I am so sorry; I did not realize that I couldn't use the materials or the logos."
   b. "I was just trying to help and get you more employees. Can we go ahead and use the brochures?"
   c. "Oh well, too late; everything is already printed and I said we would have a booth."
   d. "I think it will be okay as long as no one complains about the logos."

Code 1.12 Test Yourself: True or False Questions

2. You are an RBT and former computer graphics major who is presenting on the BACB and the field of ABA for your Intro to Psychology class. It seems to you that the BACB logo needs some work, and you decide to touch it up just a little for your presentation. Such minor modifications are not a code violation.

   True or False?

   True

   False
3. Your company asks you to make copies of a blank ABLLS-R (Assessment of Basic Language and Learning Skills-Revised) to begin an assessment for a new client. This is not a

violation since the company authorized you to make the copies.

True or False?

True

False

For correct answers, go to Appendix A

1.13 RBTs ATTEMPT TO RESOLVE ISSUES INFORMALLY WHEN POSSIBLE, WITHOUT VIOLATING CONFIDENTIALITY, BY FIRST BRINGING THE ISSUE TO THE ATTENTION OF THEIR SUPERVISOR AND THEN THE INDIVIDUAL INVOLVED. RBTs DOCUMENT THEIR EFFORTS TO ADDRESS ANY OF THESE ISSUES. IF THE MATTER CANNOT BE RESOLVED INFORMALLY, THEY REPORT IT TO THE APPROPRIATE AUTHORITY (E.G., EMPLOYER, DIRECTOR, REGULATORY AUTHORITY). IF THE MATTER MEETS THE REPORTING REQUIREMENTS OF THE BACB, RBTs MUST SUBMIT A FORMAL COMPLAINT TO THE BACB

Quick Take

"If there was potential for harm, under this Code item, you would immediately go to your supervisor or other relevant authority for advice and carefully follow that guidance."

The intent of this Code item is that RBTs should be aware of the activities of other RBTs and supervisors and be prepared to respond appropriately to remind them of the RBT Ethics Code. In the case of a *minor* incident such as entering data after a session is over instead of during the session or accepting a small gift from a client, the RBT should engage the person in a conversation (not a confrontation), bring up the ethics question, and then gauge their response. If this was just a misunderstanding or a simple error, and you are satisfied with the response, there is no reason to take the matter further, and you can consider it resolved. On the other hand, if what you observed involved a client's legal rights being violated (see RBT Codes 2.01, 2.02), or if there was potential for harm, under this Code item, you would immediately go to your supervisor or other relevant authority for advice and carefully follow that guidance. They may prep you on how to handle the issue, or they may decide to take responsibility for resolving the problem. Be sure to document (write an email or memo to the relevant authority, e.g., your supervisor, clinical director, CEO) what you saw and how you responded. In a situation where you feel that one of these individuals did not respond appropriately, your final resort is to file a Notice with the BACB.

CHALLENGE 1: You are working in a clinic setting with an RBT who often appears impatient when working with clients. One day, you observe the RBT working with a client who is having a tantrum and see him roughly escort the client to a makeshift timeout room in the corner of the room. You bring the situation to the attention of his BCBA supervisor, who happens to also be the clinical director. The clinical director assures you the issue will be resolved. However, since the initial incident, you have seen and reported two more similar incidents to the supervisor/clinical director and there appears to be no visible action taken to resolve the problem.

WHAT NOT TO DO: Assume that you have done all you can in bringing this issue to the attention of the clinical director and move on.

WHAT *TO* DO: Document your previous attempts to resolve the issue in writing, make sure you have an email paper trail of your interactions and detailed and dated notes following each interaction. All of this information should then be brought to the clinical director's supervisor.

COMMENTARY: The ethical RBT did the right thing by bringing this to the attention of the RBT's supervisor, as he was committing a serious violation that placed the client at risk. Unfortunately, her attempts were unsuccessful and required her to go up the chain of command. If still unresolved, a Notice of Alleged Violation Form could be filed with the BACB.

CHALLENGE 2: Yamilex is an RBT working at an agency that services clients in their school. Due to this environment, she rarely sees other coworkers and only sees a BCBA when they come to supervise her. She and another RBT from her agency are working in the same classroom, but Yamilex notices the other RBT is constantly late to her session. The teacher has made comments to Yamilex about the other RBT being late and wants to know who they can talk to about it. The other RBT made comments to Yamilex such as, "It's okay to be late since no one is going to know and I can still bill for the whole time."

RBT RESPONSE: Yamilex decided to talk to the RBT about her tardiness when she arrived late again for her session in the classroom, "It's kind of unprofessional to be late all the time. You know when your session starts, your client is waiting, and you need to be here. I can't keep covering for you. If there is an issue with transportation or something, then you should bring that up with your BCBA."

COMMENTARY: Yamilex should have gone to her supervisor about the possible billing fraud. This discussion should not have taken place in the classroom with the teacher present, who is already having issues with the RBT. This also took away from her training session with the client. It is the job of the supervisor to step in and discuss this with the habitually tardy RBT. Managing an RBT is not a part of Yamilex's job responsibilities.

CHALLENGE 3: You are an RBT who is working with a client in the classroom. There is another client who receives services from your agency in that classroom as well. The teacher in this classroom has been known to use methods that are not behavior analytical and often asks the RBTs to implement her methods. You noticed that the other RBT is using the teacher's "mindfulness" techniques instead of the approved behavior-reduction protocol. The other RBT tells you that they think this is more effective at decreasing the problem behavior and they plan on continuing to use mindfulness techniques in the future.

RBT RESPONSE: You decide to inform your shared supervisor about what you saw happen in the classroom and tell your supervisor that you didn't think you were supposed to implement non-behavior analytic approaches.

COMMENTARY: In ABA, we do not use methods that do not have an evidence-based backing. "Mindfulness" does not have solid behavior-analytic research to support it. This RBT was correct to bring the issue to their shared supervisor and allow the supervisor to intervene rather than the RBT attempting to correct the problem.

CHALLENGE 4: You (RBT 1) are assigned to a classroom where RBT 2, a new employee at your company, also works. The teacher consistently offers you both food from the teachers' lounge. You always decline, but today, you notice RBT 2 accepting a doughnut and eating it in the classroom.

RBT 1 RESPONSE: (pulls RBT 2 aside at the end of the day), "Hey, I am not sure if you are aware, but we are not supposed to be taking any of the food from the teacher's lounge, as it falls under our code on accepting gifts."

RBT 2 RESPONSE: "Wow, I am so sorry. I didn't know."

RBT 1 RESPONSE: "That's what I thought—just wanted to make sure to let you know."

COMMENTARY: RBT 1 was able to informally address the violation with RBT 2 without formally bringing this to the attention of the supervisor. The following is an unofficial list showing a ranked ordering of types of violations from least to most severe that can be used to give you an idea of which violations might be treated informally and which are considered serious.[3]

Ranked Ordering of Ethical Violations

These violations can be treated informally.

- Unauthorized use of copy machine
- Tardiness
- Ignorance of the RBT Ethics Code
- Accepting gifts like food or drinks from clients
- Giving gifts to clients
- Errors in discrete trial training (DTT) implementation, for example, improper prompting, reinforcement error

- - - - - - - - - - - - - - -

These are serious violations.

- Not following protocol for behavior reduction
- Faking data collection
- Implementing an unauthorized punisher (time out, response cost, etc.)
- Withholding food as an unauthorized punisher

3 This chart does not represent the thinking of the BACB or any official organization of behavior analysts.

- Lying to parents about treatment progress
- Accepting large gifts from parents (TV, cash, etc.)
- Discussing confidential client information with unauthorized individuals without consent
- Engaging in a sexual relationship with clients or supervisors
- Deliberate falsification of billing
- Abusing a client, for example, pinching, slapping, forced holding

> "If a client's legal rights are being violated or there is a potential for harm, you must take necessary action to protect the client."

More Details

This Code item is derived from the BACB Code 7.02 (a, b, c, d), which bears reading since it is more expansive in describing the sequence of events. First you determine if there is *potential for harm*, a *possible legal violation*, or a *mandatory-reporting condition.* Next, if a client's legal rights are being violated or there is potential for harm, you must take necessary action to protect the client. If the violation does not reach this level, that is, a minor issue, then try to resolve it informally. Even if you resolve an issue informally, you should still document your observations and actions. Finally, you could file a formal complaint (Notice of Alleged Violation) with the BACB if action on a serious matter is not resolved informally.

Code 1.13 Test Yourself: Multiple-Choice Questions

1. You notice another RBT is always on their phone during her sessions. The client's teacher has mentioned something to this RBT about being on the phone, but the RBT continues to use the phone. The RBT told the teacher that it's typical for therapists to be on their phones in case their supervisor contacts them. How should you respond?
   a. Apologize to the teacher for the other RBT's behavior and never take your phone out during a session.

b. Tell the teacher it is typical for RBTs to use their phones and start using your phone as well.
c. Bring the issue up with your supervisor and relay the teacher's frustrations.
d. Talk to the RBT yourself and tell her to stop using her phone during sessions.

2. You and another RBT are having issues about where to keep a client's reinforcers. After every session, you both leave the bag of reinforcers in a different spot and then have to search for it at the start of the next session. You are both becoming frustrated with each other. How should you respond?
   a. Bring your supervisor into this argument because they have time to handle this.
   b. Keep moving the reinforcers, and eventually, you will both decide on a place to keep them.
   c. Start leaving the reinforcers in the therapy rooms and hope the other clients can't find them.
   d. Get together and decide on a place that you both think could work.
3. RBT 1 witnesses RBT 2 utilizing a hold for a client whose protocol states explicitly never to use one. How should RBT 1 respond?
   a. Immediately inform the client's parent.
   b. Wait and see what happens; it may have been a misunderstanding and you do not want to intervene while RBT 2 is implementing the procedure.
   c. Address the RBT to inquire about the unauthorized hold and contact the supervisor, informing them of what is occurring.
   d. File a Notice of Alleged Violation as soon as you can.

Code 1.13 Test Yourself: True or False Questions

4. You have been training a new RBT for a couple of weeks when you observe him implement the reduction behavior protocol with the client incorrectly. When you ask him about it, he tells you that another RBT told him he was

doing it wrong. You realize this means other therapists are doing things differently and don't know how to properly implement the protocol. You tell the new RBT to ignore what the other tech said and to follow *your* original instructions and to please ignore anything else that RBT tells him. This RBT should have brought this serious issue to the supervisor.

True or False?

True

False

For correct answers, go to Appendix A

5

Section 2—Responsibility to Clients Codes 2.01–2.10

In Section 1, the BACB RBT Ethics Code emphasizes the importance of the science of behavior and the significance of your personal character as a truthful, honest person. In Section 2, our code emphasizes your responsibility to the clients that you serve. Our top priority is that you respect and support the rights of clients, both legal and in simple everyday preferences. To make this more accessible, we have provided a list of commonly accepted clients' rights (Code 2.01) in this chapter. The code further prompts RBTs to take action if necessary to protect clients' rights (Code 2.02) by contacting the relevant authorities and documenting your efforts. Related to this is your obligation as an RBT not to discriminate against clients on any basis (Code 2.03).

Giving gifts as a sign of appreciation is common across many cultures, but in behavior analysis, accepting a gift from a client can lead to a multiple relationship (Code 1.06). This then leads to a personal decision that affects behavior-analytic treatment adversely. We discuss this extensively in this code and provide many examples of where gift giving has gone wrong.

Another cultural feature that can impact client services is social media and the internet. Sharing photos and information on Facebook and other platforms has become a part of daily life, so much so that when people embark on a professional career, they feel they want to publicly share those details, too. This is not allowed by Code 2.05 because of the dangers of predators on the internet and dark net who can capture and manipulate this information for their own dangerous and perverse purposes. Somewhat related to this is the ubiquity of recording almost everything in our culture, from sports events to birthdays, but we have no right to record clients or staff at work unless written consent is given from each person.

Codes 2.05, 2.06, 2.07, 2.08, and 2.09 all have to do with protecting client information from those who do not legitimately need access to it. RBTs are a significant part of this system since they have such close contact with confidential material. RBTs are warned about exposing confidential material about clients on social media (2.05), gaining permission for any recordings (2.06), using only relevant identifying information in their emails and reports (2.07), only sharing confidential information with those who need to know (2.08), and, finally, never disclosing confidential information without consent (2.09).

One final piece of protection of confidentiality is that any data or records must be created and ultimately disposed of according to laws and regulations, many of which are issued by the Health Insurance Portability and Accountability Act of 1996 (HIPAA).

2.01 RBTs SUPPORT THE LEGAL RIGHTS AND PREFERENCES OF CLIENTS

Quick Take

In order to *support the legal rights of clients*, it is first necessary to understand what those rights are. This may depend on the state where you are practicing, so you may want to go to your state government website and search for "Bill of Rights of Persons Who Are Developmentally Disabled." This can be a very long list, more than we can cover completely, but here are some basics related to client rights.

Clients Have a Right to . . .

> *"Given the role of RBTs in the chain of behavioral services, this would mean that you would promote the rights of your clients and assist them in achieving their preferences."*

- Self-determination
- Training to maximize their potential to lead independent and productive lives
- Minimal use of restraint and seclusion and least restrictive conditions
- Individual dignity, personal liberty, pursuit of happiness, and humane care
- Religious freedom
- Social interaction and community activities
- Physical exercise and recreational opportunities
- Be free from harm, isolation, excessive medication, abuse, and neglect
- Consent to or refuse treatment
- Vote in public elections
- Unrestricted communications
- Possession and use of their own clothing
- Medication only by order of a physician. Medication may not be used as punishment or for the convenience of staff, and it should not substitute for a behavior analysis plan
- An exam by a physician to eliminate organic causes before a treatment plan to eliminate problem behavior is implemented

In addition, if you are to *support client preferences*, you would need to know what those are. You or the BCBA should have conducted preference assessments prior to any behavior plans being proposed. These choices might include choice of clothing, food and drink, living arrangements, friends, daily scheduling, entertainment, recreation, and more.

A key word in this Code item is "support," and it is important to understand what this means when it comes to *supporting* client rights and preferences. Given the role of RBTs in the chain of behavioral services, this would mean that you would promote the rights of your clients and assist them in achieving their preferences. You should argue for certain rights if it appears these rights are being challenged. Being an advocate and being outspoken on behalf of your clients is essential to providing support.

CHALLENGE 1: In one of the classrooms where you are working, the teacher frequently uses punishment with the students. When your client engages in problem behavior, you implement the approved protocol, which does not include punishment. Today, when you arrived at your session, you saw the teacher withholding your client's lunch because she was engaging in problem behavior. You found out from the aide that the teacher has been withholding the client's lunch consistently when a therapist is not present, and now the teacher has asked you to do the same because it is *her* classroom.

RBT RESPONSE: "I'm sorry, but I am restricted to following the approved treatment protocol my supervisor has given me. If you have any concerns, please speak to my supervisor. It would be unethical for me to withhold my client's lunch."

TEACHER RESPONSE: "I don't see why withholding lunch is a problem; this is *my* classroom, and I have *my* rules."

COMMENTARY: Withholding a client's lunch certainly violates your client's rights, and a situation like this should be addressed immediately. This RBT did the right thing by letting the teacher know she would not withhold the client's lunch. The next step would be contacting both the supervisor and caregivers to let them know what has been happening and try to see a resolution.

CHALLENGE 2: A dialogue between two RBTs about a client follows.

RBT 1: "Hey, how was Jackson today?"

RBT 2: "We had the same problems we have been having because I was denying him access to a toy he was stimming on (using for self-stimulatory behavior). I hate to see him do that."

RBT 1: "I think we are going to need to talk to the BCBA about this. Jackson's behaviors are increasing in every session. How was he outside?"

RBT 2: "I didn't take him outside. He kept asking, but I didn't feel like dealing with him once we got out there. He has been having tantrums, oops, I mean engaging in emotional outbursts, when we go outside. I guess this is because I won't let him take that toy outside either."

RBT 1: "Hmm, well, I understand that Jackson's behaviors are increasing, and we aren't sure why, but we can't ethically deny him access to playing outside because he *might* engage in problem behaviors. I think we should talk to our supervisor about what's been going on."

COMMENTARY: The second RBT was not implementing the client's programs correctly and decided to start denying the client access to outside play because she didn't want to deal with the problem behavior. Access to recreation is a client's right. Treatment changes like this should never be made by the RBT without obtaining prior approval from the supervisor.

CHALLENGE 3: In a clinic setting where you are RBT, clients come for the day and are scheduled to participate in a variety of group activities. Sophia engages in high rates of problem behaviors during the activities. Your supervisor recommends an FR1 schedule of edible reinforcement for compliance with any task. This works at first, but unfortunately, the RBT quickly runs out of the edibles supplied by the caregiver, and

Sophia often spends the remaining hours sitting in the corner of the room, refusing to comply with any instruction.

RBT RESPONSE: "I am having some issues with this intervention. It seems to work at first, but once we run out of food, I am not sure what I am supposed to do."

BCBA RESPONSE: "Food is the only thing that she is motivated by, and we can only use what her parents provide, so there is really not much we can do."

RBT RESPONSE: "But sometimes she sits in the corner for nearly an hour until she gets picked up. Is there anything else that we can be doing?"

BCBA RESPONSE: "The results from our paired-choice preference assessment showed that Sophia only selected edible items. Even when presented with two tangible items, she would not select anything. We cannot control her interests that are very selective, so we just need to do what we can with what we have."

COMMENTARY: Here it appears the BCBA has given up, thus restricting the client's ability to interact with peers, engage in activities, and receive training to maximize independent living. As the client is now spending extended periods isolating herself in the corner of the room, she is no longer receiving effective treatment. Although the RBT's initial attempt has not been effective, a second attempt with offering possible solutions may be more effective (for example, re-assessing stimuli used in previous assessments, consulting with parents on preferred activities at home,

> *"To live up to this expectation, RBTs may ask themselves upon reviewing the client's situation, "How would I like to be treated?" Put another way, "How would I like my brother or sister to be treated?"*

and modifying the current intervention or schedule of activities). If still unsuccessful, the RBT should then bring this matter to the BCBA's supervisor.

More Details

This Code item elevates the role of the RBT from a technician who does what they are told to a thinking and caring RBT who is watching out for the client's best interest at the macro level. They ask questions such as, "Is this behavior program in my client's best interest, or is it simply the parents' preference?" "Should we be using this contingency with this client since he has a right to communication?" In the world of human services, this type of questioning and oversight are usually delegated to social workers, who work hard to protect their clients' freedom, dignity, and humane care. By including this item in our RBT Ethics Code, we are saying that we value the position of the RBTs because they have the greatest access to the clients day to day. RBTs know more about client concerns, what rights might be disregarded, and client preferences. To live up to this expectation, RBTs may ask themselves upon reviewing the client's situation, "How would I like to be treated?" Put another way, "How would I like my brother or sister to be treated?" This person-centered approach compels RBTs to be constantly on their toes, aware of any violations of client's rights or infringement on their preferences.

Code 2.01 Test Yourself: Multiple-Choice Questions

1. An instructor who does not believe in ABA therapy is the lead teacher for a class where you have a client. Your client has good verbal skills and has told you that he doesn't like to be touched. All of his therapists are aware of the need to reduce any physical contact with the client. This was communicated to the teacher, but when you arrived at your session, you saw the teacher was holding the client

down, "Because he was noncompliant." How should you respond?

a. "Maybe you shouldn't be working with young children—it looks like they upset you."
b. "I already told you that he doesn't like to be touched, and it looks like you are just touching him as a punishment."
c. "He has told us that he prefers to be not be touched, and we should respect that. I'm sure my supervisor would love to show you the protocol we use when he engages in property destruction."
d. "Well, this doesn't seem like the best idea to me, but it is your classroom and I will respect your opinion."

Code 2.01 Test Yourself: True or False Questions

2. The reinforcers for Akari are typically light-up toys that make sounds. Akari engages in problem behaviors frequently during nonpreferred tasks, but he will work for the light-up toys. The next time you arrive at your RBT session, the teacher tells you that you can no longer use those toys because they are too loud, and she thinks they are annoying. You decide that it is the teacher's classroom and she is allowed to choose. Respect for client preferences only matters when you are working in an ABA clinic.

   True or False?

   True

   False

3. A client with severe eczema engages in frequent scratching. Your client prefers to apply his lotion by himself, but it takes him about 15 minutes. Your client's class is trying to leave to go to recess, but he is still putting his lotion on. Under Code 2.01, you know that it's important to respect your client's preferences.

   True or False?

   True

   False

4. A 16-year-old client who is working on social skills goals with you has informed you on multiple occasions that he does not want therapy and that having an RBT at school with him causes other students to pick on him. Since he isn't an adult, Code 2.01 doesn't apply to him but applies to his parents, who do want him to have therapy.

   True or False?

   True

   False

For correct answers, go to Appendix A

FOR FURTHER READING

Here are some websites that may be useful in learning about the basic rights of clients.

http://apd.myflorida.com/training/docs/bill-of-rights-2008.pdf
www.leg.state.fl.us/Statutes/index.cfm?App_mode=Display_Statute&URL=0300-0399/0381/Sections/0381.026.html

2.02 IF RBTs BECOME AWARE THAT A CLIENT'S LEGAL RIGHTS ARE BEING VIOLATED, OR IF THERE IS RISK OF HARM, RBTs MUST TAKE THE NECESSARY ACTION TO PROTECT THE CLIENT. THIS INCLUDES BUT IS NOT LIMITED TO: (1) CONTACTING RELEVANT AUTHORITIES; (2) FOLLOWING ORGANIZATIONAL POLICIES; (3) CONSULTING WITH THEIR SUPERVISOR; AND (4) DOCUMENTING THEIR EFFORTS TO ADDRESS THE MATTER

Quick Take

This Code item is directly related to Code 1.13. It requires you to 1) be aware of conditions surrounding your client, 2) remain constantly on the lookout for any violations of their legal rights (see Code 2.01 for a long list of these), and 3) stay aware of the

> *"Although it is not written this way, we think that the first thing you would do is reach out to your supervisor for advice."*

client's physical and psychological condition so there are no apparent or potential risks of harm. Although it is not written this way, we think that the first thing you would do, per Code 1.13, is reach out to your supervisor for advice. If there is no supervisor available, you may need to contact relevant authorities such as the clinical director of your organization, Child Protective Services, the Health Department, or perhaps even the Sherriff's Department. If there is time to look up organizational policies (which might describe a different sequence of decision-making), you would definitely want to do this, since it could change your action plan. As in Code 1.13, for your own protection, you should document what you observed and what you did.

CHALLENGE 1: As you approach the front door of your client's home, you see that the door is partway open. You call out, "Hello, anyone home?" No one answers, so you speak louder and repeat, "Hello, is anyone here?" There is still no response, so you head to your client's bedroom and find him sitting on the floor rocking and playing with a toy.

RBT RESPONSE: You determine that a 4-year-old, nonverbal child being left alone poses a significant personal risk, so you immediately call your supervisor. She says she will be right over and to call 911 and ask them what to do next.

COMMENTARY: This RBT was right to act immediately to ensure the safety of the client. Always make sure to call your supervisor to get help rather than attempting to solve the problem by yourself. This scenario can quickly turn into a life-or-death situation.

CHALLENGE 2: You are working in the client's home with a child who is engaging in aggression. As you are implementing the blocking protocol, the father walks in and tells you, "Don't be afraid to hit him back when he hits you like that."

RBT RESPONSE: "That is not something that I can do. The protocol involves just blocking the aggression by putting an arm up and waiting until he is calm."

FATHER: "I'm just saying, if it's something you want to do, I'm alright with it."

RBT RESPONSE: "We are not allowed to do anything like that."

COMMENTARY: The RBT both denied the use of any physical punishment as well as informing the father of the approved protocol. Next, the supervisor should be notified, as it appears the father could use more information and training on his child's treatment.

CHALLENGE 3: Over the last two weeks, you have noticed that your client's hair has not been washed, he's wearing the same clothes every day, and his lunch has only consisted of half a sandwich. Your client has also missed school on many days. Mom has asked you to not mention the child's hygiene to anyone, and she said that she might have to stop services because they are getting too expensive.

RBT RESPONSE: You decide to not tell anyone what you have been observing because his mother knows best and you don't want to lose this client.

COMMENTARY: Actually, the RBT should have immediately contacted her supervisor to discuss this situation. The concern here should be primarily for the client's welfare, and Child Protective Services may need to be called.

CHALLENGE 4: The client in this case is a little girl who has recently been put on a gluten-free diet by her pediatrician for medical reasons. Her father has given you (as the RBT) and the rest of the team a list of the foods Skyler needs to avoid. One day, the new stepmother dropped Skyler off with a lunch including a sandwich and a cookie.

RBT RESPONSE: "It looks like Skyler has bread in her lunch today. My supervisor told me we were not allowed to give her anything with gluten in it. Is this still correct?"

STEPMOTHER: "That doctor is a joke. Look, she's fine, I let her have bread all the time and she looks pretty healthy to me, even with the occasional diarrhea. Her dad is overreacting. This whole thing is ridiculous, I don't like the way he pampers her all the time."

RBT RESPONSE: "Okay, we'll allow the bread if you are sure that Skyler will be fine. We will see you in a few hours."

COMMENTARY: Here the RBT tried to do the right thing by first addressing the concern with the client's mother (who was no longer living in the home). However, the RBT should have gone to her supervisor for help with the situation. A meeting with the family is needed to develop a consistent plan. Gluten intolerance can have serious effects on some individuals; if they don't stay on the diet, symptoms can include diarrhea, bloating, headaches, and more.

> *"You will need to be aware of a client's right to dignity and humane care as well as religious freedom and a right to exercise and recreation."*

More Details

RBTs are the frontline protectors of clients' safety, welfare, and legal rights (see Code 2.01) since they spend so much with them. You would be the first to notice if a client had a bruise or an injury or was crying or withdrawn. This Code is a prompt to be on your toes looking out for anything unusual and to be prepared to take action. With regard to their legal rights, you will need to be aware of a client's right to dignity and humane care as well as religious freedom and a right to exercise and recreation. There are circumstances where these rights are taken away as consequences for behavior (we would consider this punishment), and that would be considered a violation of a client's rights. Another right that clients have is the right to have a physician conduct an exam to rule out a biological cause of behavior before a behavior plan is put in place. Related to this, the client has a right to have any needed medications prescribed by a physician, who will specify that the prescriptions are not to be used as punishment, for the convenience of staff, or to replace a behavior plan.

This Code also emphasizes that RBTs *must take action* if they become aware of a threat to their client's safety or to their legal rights. The action depends on the risk of harm or severity of legal-rights violation and should be proportionate. For example, if you observe a client being deprived of recreation or exercise, you would speak to your supervisor; if you see bruising on your client and observe the parent in a rage with a belt in his or her hand, you would call Child Protective Services and then call your supervisor. If you observed drug paraphernalia in the home, you would call 911 or the Sheriff's Office and then inform your supervisor.

When you are first hired by a company, you should spend some time with the policy and procedures manual so that you fully understand the organization's policies. These policies and procedures may guide your actions in situations such as those described previously. Finally, as in Code 1.13, it is important to make a habit of documenting any observations and/or actions that you take. If you meet with your supervisor and raise a concern about a client, be sure to follow this up with a verbatim account of what was discussed. A common phrase in legal circles is, "If it is not in writing, it does not exist."

Code 2.02 Test Yourself: Multiple-Choice Questions

1. An RBT arrived at a session and saw the client's teacher force-feeding him. The client, Oliver, was clearly requesting "all done," but the teacher continued to put food in his mouth and then hold it shut. When the RBT asked the teacher what was happening, the teacher said that Oliver was "being bad" and needed to eat his lunch. How should the RBT have responded?
   a. Walk out of the classroom and wait for lunch to be over—the RBT would not want to be liable for this.
   b. The RBT should tell the teacher, "I am here now. I can help prompt Oliver to eat as we should be doing with the feeding program."
   c. Ignore what was happening and just take the food from the teacher and start the session.
   d. Inform the teacher that the RBT's supervisor would be contacted because force feeding is going against what the client has requested. The supervisor will advise the RBT on how to proceed.
2. In your RBT job, you are working with a client in his classroom where there are three other students. His teacher has absolutely no experience working with young children or children with special needs. The teacher plays videos all day and then sits in her office until it's time for the students to go home. She does not let the children play with toys, and she has stopped taking the class to the playground. Recently, she told you that your client can no longer go to his special area classes (music, P.E., art, etc.) even though these are all listed in his IEP. The teacher doesn't like it that an aide has to go with you to handle this client because this leaves the remainder of the class with her. How should you respond?
   a. Say, "We are going to go anyway, so get over it."
   b. Say, "I would like to see you try to stop me. This is in the plan."

c. Say, "I am going to contact my supervisor and see if she knows if something changed. Until then, I need to follow my protocol and take him."
d. Say, "Oh, um, okay; I'm sure it won't hurt him to miss it this once."

3. Your client has a history of lying, fabricating stories, and falsely accusing people of various offenses. One day the client shows you a burn on his arm and tells you his parents burned him. How do you respond?
   a. Contact your supervisor and make a report to Child Protective Services.
   b. Assume that this is a lie because you know this client has a history of lying behavior.
   c. Ask his parents about it and see if they respond suspiciously.
   d. Wait and see if he brings it up again.

Code 2.02 Test Yourself: True or False Questions

4. Another student in your client's classroom receives services from another RBT in your agency. You observe the RBT use a restraint on her client because she was apparently frustrated, as the magnitude of the client's behavior did not meet criteria for the use of restraint. As you are unaware of the client's programming and unsure if this RBT actually violated the protocol, you do not need to report to the supervisor. This is the correct thing to do ethically.

   True or False?
   True
   False

5. While working with a client at school, you are in P.E. class. Your client has been engaging in the game independently and is engaging with peers. Your client tells you that she is tired and wants to sit down and not play the game

anymore. You decide it would be okay for her to take a break for a bit. This is the ethical thing to do.

True or False?

True

False

For correct answers, go to Appendix A

2.03 WHEN PROVIDING SERVICES, RBTs DO NOT DISCRIMINATE AGAINST, DEMEAN, OR HARASS INDIVIDUALS OR GROUPS ON THE BASIS OF AGE, GENDER, RACE, CULTURE, ETHNICITY, NATIONAL ORIGIN, RELIGION, SEXUAL ORIENTATION, DISABILITY, LANGUAGE, SOCIOECONOMIC STATUS, OR ANY OTHER BASIS FORBIDDEN BY LAW. RBTs RECOGNIZE THEIR OWN LIMITATIONS AND OBTAIN THE PROPER TRAINING, CONSULTATION, OR SUPERVISION WHEN PROVIDING BEHAVIOR TECHNICIAN SERVICES TO PROTECTED INDIVIDUALS OR GROUPS

> "Being prejudicial in your treatment of clients (or observing it in other behavior analysts) is a form of bias that is not acceptable in our field."

Quick Take

This Code item includes two important concepts for practicing RBTs. First, it is imperative that you not discriminate against your clients in any way for any reason, and second, that you recognize your boundaries of competence. If you are required to provide service with a new client population or behavior problem, you will need to find someone (presumably your supervisor) to train you. Being prejudicial in your treatment of clients (or observing it in other behavior analysts) is a form of bias that is not acceptable in our field. Examples of this are being intolerant of others' beliefs or behavior; showing favoritism toward some clients as opposed to others based on skin color, age, or sex; or treating some clients differently because of their culture or ethnicity.

When you were a RBT-in-training, you probably worked with one type of client, such as young children with ASD or teens with behavior disorders. The company that hired you should have discussed your experience with you in some detail and then described the kinds of clients they served. This was your chance to say, "I haven't worked with teenagers before, but I am willing to learn. Is there someone here who can train me?" Supervisors are actually cautioned not to delegate responsibilities to their supervisees that the supervisees cannot handle (see Code 5.03). Supervisors are required by their Code 5.04 to provide you with the proper training. Any time you are learning a new skill, you should receive feedback and reinforcement throughout the process until you are ready to perform on your own (see Code 5.06).

CHALLENGE 1: You are providing services to a family whose first language is Spanish. The client's parents speak little English, and your company doesn't employ very many Spanish speakers. Your supervisor needs to have a parental consent form translated and asks you for help.

RBT RESPONSE: You decide not to translate the consent form because you feel the parents should be able to communicate in English with English-speaking therapists. You press the parents to sign the English version of the consent form by holding out a pen and pointing to the signature line.

COMMENTARY: This RBT is violating Code 2.03 and discriminating against a family because of their first language. She is discriminating against the parents' right to know what is happening with their child, and this will affect their ability to make informed decisions for the child.

CHALLENGE 2: One of your clients will be starting training sessions in the home. You are excited because you have only met the dad and not the mother, and today, you are expecting both parents to be present during your visit. Upon arriving at the home, you become aware that this client doesn't have a mother. His two parents are *Dad* and *Daddy*. Due to your personal beliefs, you do not implement the training programs with both parents, nor do you speak to both dads. Noticing that there is not data recorded for both parents, your supervisor asks what is happening with the training sessions.

RBT RESPONSE: Tell your supervisor that you feel that the client's parents should not be receiving treatment. You feel that your agency should not offer services to this *family*.

COMMENTARY: You are an RBT representing your field and your agency. Even though you are a person who has rights, while providing therapy, you have to put any personal beliefs aside to ensure the highest quality of care for your client. You can certainly have a discussion with your supervisor about your beliefs, but you work for this company to serve clients and implement treatment. By not doing the training properly (with both parents) and therefore discriminating against this family, you are violating the code of ethics.

CHALLENGE 3: An RBT where you are working has made previous comments about how much she enjoys working with young clients. The company you both work for promotes a training program that involves having RBTs train with clients of all ages to ensure a well-rounded experience. This RBT has now been assigned to work with an older client, and you often hear her complaining about how much she dislikes this and wishes they would take her off the case.

WHAT NOT TO SAY: "Clearly you don't enjoy working with older clients; I don't even know why you are in this job. People of all ages need help and the way you are acting is incredibly offensive. You are giving ABA a bad name and should really consider looking elsewhere for a job."

WHAT *TO* SAY: "You know, I didn't have much experience working with older clients before I came here. I never really saw myself working with this population, but once I started, I was amazed at how much I enjoyed it. It was tough for me to adjust to at first, so if you ever need some help, I'm always here to talk."

COMMENTARY: This RBTs frustration may be a result of her limited experience, so your empathy and assistance might be enough to help get her on track. A combative response in a situation like this will most likely not help. Showing understanding and offering assistance might be all that is needed. Another thing you could stress to the other RBT is that by working with different age groups, she will expand her skill set and give her more job opportunities down the road. However, if your attempts to have the RBT be more open-minded do not have an effect on the RBT's discriminatory statements, you should bring this to the attention of your supervisor.

> *"The Americans with Disabilities Act (ADA) of 1990 prohibits discrimination against 'a person who has a physical or mental impairment that substantially limits one or more major life activities'."*

More Details

Discrimination against clients on any basis is abhorrent and unacceptable in applied behavior analysis. This position is directly in line with federal law. Title VII of the 1964 Civil Rights Act makes it illegal to "Discriminate against someone on the basis of race, color, religion, national origin, or sex." In addition, the Americans with Disabilities Act (ADA) of 1990 prohibits discrimination against "A person who has a physical or mental impairment that substantially limits one or more major life activities, a person who has a history or record of such an impairment, or a person who is perceived by others as having such an impairment." Another legal right of clients is covered by the Individuals with Disabilities Education Act (IDEA), which requires public schools to provide children with disabilities a "Free appropriate public education in the least restrictive environment appropriate to their individual needs." As you can see, keeping track of all the legal rights of clients is no small task and could require some reading and research on your part.

Revealing your limitations to your supervisor can be personally threatening; it makes you vulnerable to criticism and could hinder your advancement in an organization. However, if this is what it takes for you to receive proper training to handle difficult situations with clients, then it will be worthwhile in the long run. In the short run, your clients will benefit since they will receive what is required by BACB Code 2.09, that is, the "Right to effective treatment." While the *right to effective treatment* is not written in federal law, it is a bedrock assumption of applied behavior analysis. It was passed by a resolution of the Association for Behavior Analysis in 1988 and published in the *Journal of Applied Behavior Analysis* that same year.

Code 2.03 Test Yourself: Multiple-Choice Question

1. Recently, your supervisor informed you that you will be working with a new client who engages in pica. You have never worked with a client with this disorder before. How should you respond?
   a. Do some research on your own on pica. If you read articles about pica, you should be able to provide treatment.
   b. Talk to other RBTs about their experience with pica to gather information on what interventions they have used.

c. Inform your supervisor that you do not have experience with pica but that you are interested to learn and would like some training and mentoring to teach you to work with this problem.
d. Nothing; just wait and see what happens when you start working with the client. It may not be as hard as you think.

Code 2.03 Test Yourself: True or False Questions

2. The school play is coming up, and you have been working with your client on where to stand on stage and when to sit down. Her original place was at the front with the other children, but the teacher saw her engaging in stereotypy (hand flapping) and immediately moved her to the back where no one could see her. You discuss this change with the teacher and request to have your client moved back to the front of the stage. You say it's not fair that the client was moved due to the hand flapping. Your response was an appropriate ethical action under Code 2.03.
   True or False?
   True
   False
3. A young client who is bilingual has parents who speak limited English. You often have difficulty communicating with them at drop-off and pick-up at the clinic. You do not want to offend the parents, so you often appear as if you are understanding what they are saying by head nodding, smiling, and providing a very basic description of what happened in the session. This approach is a violation of Code 2.03.
   True or False?
   True
   False

For correct answers, go to Appendix A

2.04 RBTs DO NOT ACCEPT GIFTS FROM OR GIVE GIFTS TO CLIENTS

> *"We believe that this is the type of relationship RBTs should have with the families they serve: Friendly but not Friends."*

Quick Take

The intent of Code 2.04 is to reduce the possibility of the RBT becoming too friendly with clients, thus creating a multiple relationship (Code 1.06) and resulting in impaired professional judgment.

Friends exchange gifts on certain holidays, for birthdays, and on special occasions. In a *professional* relationship, the patient just says, "Thank you so much, doctor. I really appreciate you working me in today. I was really feeling miserable when I woke up this morning." And the MD says, "You are quite welcome, Mrs. Miller. We value our long-term patients and will always be here for you." We believe that this is the type of relationship RBTs, and BCBAs as well, should have with the families they serve: Friendly but not Friends.

Accepting gifts from clients, regardless of the size or amount, breaks that professional bond and sets the stage for possible manipulation of the judgment of the RBT and perhaps the whole behavior analysis team. An offer of a "free" trip to Aspen for a ski vacation—"You can work with Charlie while we are on the slopes, and we'll give you Thursday and Friday morning off so you can ski"—is a truly exciting offer but off limits for RBTs because it is an example of an extravagant "gift" that may turn out to be little more than a bribe attempt in the long run where the parents will ask for a favor down the road.

Needless to say, RBTs should not be giving gifts to clients or their parents since this also represents a "friends" connection, also known as a multiple relationship.

We believe the intent of this code item is to disallow all multiple relationships, including not giving gifts to your supervisor or to a teacher in the classroom where you work with your client. You may, of course, give a gift to another RBT since there is no supervisory relationship there. If you give a gift to an RBT, you should be sensitive about whether there are other RBTs who also work with you who could have their feelings hurt if they do not receive a gift. You may give a small gift to a former client once you are no longer working with that family.

There is one exception to the "no gifting" rule. A handmade card from a child or DD client is considered an innocent expression of appreciation with no ulterior motive. A handmade card was not purchased from Hallmark and has no street value and therefore is not a "gift."

CHALLENGE 1: You have been working with client for a while and have become very close to her family. The client's mother also serves as her teacher at the school. The mother has shared personal stories and some private information with you. During your session, the class is celebrating your client's birthday. The mother tells you to take a cupcake and snacks because you are practically family.

RBT RESPONSE: Only take a cupcake and not the other snacks. It is your client's birthday, and the mother told you to take the cupcake, and you don't want to appear rude.

COMMENTARY: While it can be fun to have a cupcake with your client's class, it would still be unethical for you to take a cupcake or any of the snacks. Those are still gifts, and the best thing to do is to just say, "No thank you" and move on.

CHALLENGE 2: The company you work for has a long history of giving gifts to the teachers and classroom aides of the clients. The company believes that the giving of small gifts helps build a relationship with the teachers. Your supervisor has asked you to take a gift to your client's teacher (you don't feel comfortable about this, but everyone else at the company is doing it, so you are unsure of what to do).

WHAT *NOT* TO DO: You give the gift anyway. You figure that if something was wrong with giving gifts, then your agency wouldn't do it. You also don't want to get in trouble with your supervisor. Besides, your supervisor said that if you didn't take the gift to the teacher, she would find someone else to do this for her.

WHAT *TO* DO: Let the supervisor know you do not feel comfortable providing the teacher with a gift, as you are aware that your company should not be giving them gifts.

COMMENTARY: It's going to feel awkward and uncomfortable to tell your supervisor, "No; it doesn't feel right to me," but it's important to know that supervisors are also held to the code. This supervisor was violating the code by asking you take the gift to the teacher, but as the RBT, you need to uphold the code and be able to tell your supervisor when they are doing something wrong.

CHALLENGE 3: It is Christmas time, and you are packing up and getting ready to leave a home session when the parent walks out with a gift bag in hand. She says, "We just want you to know how much we appreciate all that you do for our family. Thank you so much for everything you have done; we want you to have this."

RBT RESPONSE: You decide to take the present because you don't want to hurt their feelings. It was only a $10 gift card, so it's not like it was that expensive.

> *"Across the globe, and throughout history, gifting has played a central role in strengthening our international and interpersonal relationships."*[1]

1 www.theatlantic.com/sponsored/hennessy-2018/what-gifting-rituals-around-globe-reveal-about-human-nature/2044/

COMMENTARY: Holidays always present a difficult time for RBTs when it comes to gift giving. One way to help reduce these uncomfortable situations is to give families notice ahead of time informing them of why you cannot accept gifts. This RBT needed to stay strong and thank them for the thought, but it would be unethical to accept the gift. When in doubt, just say "No."

More Details

Gifting is essentially a cultural practice that has the specific aim of strengthening the bonds between giver and receiver. That goal is at cross-purposes with the intent of our RBT Code 2.04, which is to ensure that our behavior analysts deal fairly and impartially with each and every client and their family. Accepting even a small gift erodes that independence and opens the door to favoritism by the RBT toward the client family.

"Across the globe, and throughout history, gifting has played a central role in strengthening our international and interpersonal relationships." It is the custom in Asian countries such as China, Vietnam, and Singapore to exchange red envelopes filled with cash as a way to welcome the Lunar New Year and spread good fortune among friends and relatives. Bringing a housewarming gift to a couple with a new home meant, literally, in ancient times, delivering actual firewood since everyone cooked and kept themselves warm using a hearth. Offering a gift and having it rejected multiple times is considered "proper etiquette" in many Asian countries. Regardless of the culture, "giving is almost never a truly selfless act, since reciprocity of some kind is expected," says Dr. Michael Laver, history department chair at the Rochester Institute of Technology. Marcel Mauss, a French sociologist, argues that, "Social bonds are reinforced by these mutual exchanges of gifts . . . in theory such gifts are voluntary but in fact they are given and repaid under obligation."[2]

2 M. Mauss, *The Gift: The Form and Reason for Exchange in Archaic Societies*, WW Norton Co, New York, 2000.

In this historic and worldwide context, we can see why a ban on gifts makes sense for professionals. Receiving a gift sets up an obligation for reciprocation that puts the RBT in the position of having at some point to "pay back" the giver in some way. This payback might be in the form of extra treatment at no charge, looking the other way if the parent abuses the child, or giving the child rides to the clinic or school.

Code 2.04 Test Yourself: Multiple-Choice Questions

1. On a scorching hot summer day, you and your client come inside from playing outside. The client's mother offers you a bottle of water. How should you respond?
   a. Grab the bottle eagerly because it is hot, and you deserve water.
   b. Take the water and thank the mother for being so considerate.
   c. Tell the mother no and that if she wants to continue services, she won't offer you anything else.
   d. Thank her for her hospitality, but you brought your own water bottle and are all set.
2. Arriving at work, you notice that a gift has been placed on your workstation. A coworker informs you that the parent of one of your clients asked him to bring it to you. How do you respond?
   a. Take the gift. Because you were not the one who actually accepted the gift, this would not be a violation.
   b. Throw it away. By not actually keeping the gift, you are not violating the code.
   c. Arrange to return the gift to the parent and remind them of why you are unable to accept it.
   d. Check and see what the gift is. If it does not cost more than $20, it is okay to keep it.

Code 2.04 Test Yourself: True or False Questions

3. It is February 14, and your client gives you a hand-made valentine. It is okay to accept this "gift" under Code 2.04.

True or False?
True
False

4. Today is your client's birthday and you want to give him a little gift to celebrate. You select a small toy from the store that costs less than $10 and give it to him. Since it is less than the limit under 2.04, this is acceptable.
   True or False?
   True
   False

5. You are working with a client whom you see only in school. When you arrive, he is already waiting. He gives you a gift and says, "Happy Birthday!" You do not want to make him upset by not taking it, so you keep the gift and thank him. Keeping the gift is allowed under 2.04.
   True or False?
   True
   False

For correct answers, go to Appendix A

FOR FURTHER READING

Mauss, M. (2000). *The Gift: The Form and Reason for Exchange in Archaic Societies*. New York: WW Norton Co.
www.theatlantic.com/sponsored/hennessy-2018/what-gifting-rituals-around-globe-reveal-about-human-nature/2044/

2.05 RBTs MAY NOT SHARE IDENTIFYING INFORMATION ABOUT CLIENTS ON SOCIAL MEDIA. THEY MUST AVOID CREATING SITUATIONS WHERE SUCH INFORMATION COULD BE SHARED BY OTHERS, INCLUDING, BUT NOT LIMITED TO, WRITTEN INFORMATION, PHOTOS, OR VIDEOS

Quick Take

We have become an oversharing culture, where the norm is that nearly everyone has a Facebook, Instagram, Twitter account, or

> *"Even the most innocent shot can be manipulated to create revolting pornographic images of your child."*[3]

all three plus more, and social media has become *the way* that individuals communicate with friends and family. These virtual relationships bind people together with shared experiences but are also used to create an online persona: "Look at me; I'm a foodie and here's what I had for dinner last night," "Having a great time hiking in the Rocky Mountains," "Here I am hard at work; I'm a *behavior* therapist now, and I work with kids and change their lives. Here is a pic of my latest success, Margie, who is now talking up a storm." Sharing a photo of a cute child seems so innocent and will surely impress your friends, but this is not a good idea.

The intent of Code 2.05 is to try to eliminate the possibility of a child client or DD adolescent or adult being exposed to identity thieves, predators, or pedophiles on the internet who may manipulate and share the photos or, worse, may then try to find them and do them harm. RBTs, and of course parents, should be aware that there are closed groups on Facebook where simple photos of children can be altered by sick, perverted people who use and post for the purpose of sexualizing the children in the photos. Such images have become a ruthless, malicious commodity on the dark web. For all of these reasons, RBTs are not allowed to share information about their child clients on the internet or social media.

CHALLENGE 1: Scrolling through a social media website, you notice that an RBT who works at your agency is posting a picture of her client's school. This RBT's post describes working with students at the school with autism and how rewarding her job is. Then the post talks about the client's problem behavior and how emotionally exhausting the job can be.

3 Accessed at: www.kidspot.com.au/parenting/teenager/cybersafety/what-predators-look-for-when-you-post-photos-of-your-children-online/news-story/9fea05351fdb8ab8c6bdea6acd8bfe60

RBT RESPONSE: You see the RBT the next day and tell her, "I saw your post yesterday. I just learned that we aren't allowed to post about our clients on social media. I was able to figure out who you were talking about in your post and others would be, too, so it would probably be best to take it down."

COMMENTARY: Social media is growing rapidly and has become ever present in our society. There are going to be people who post about their clients and the work that they are doing, but if you see something like this that reveals identifying information about a client, it's important to speak to them about removing this from the social media page where it appears.

CHALLENGE 2: Another RBT who is your Facebook friend does not work at your company but often posts about autism and ABA. One day you see a picture of her and a child with the caption, "So grateful to get to work with such an amazing girl; she has made so much progress since starting ABA. I can't wait to see her continue to learn and grow."

RBT 1 RESPONSE: (Sends private message). "Hey, I know you probably meant well with your last post, but I wanted to let you know that it appears to be in violation of one of our codes."

RBT 2 RESPONSE: "I talked to my supervisor and she told me it was fine. Plus, her parents know, so I don't see what the problem is."

RBT 1 RESPONSE: "Regardless of parental consent, it is still a violation of your client's privacy. Take a look at 2.05 in the RBT Ethics Code and you'll see what I'm talking about."

COMMENTARY: Clearly the supervisor misinformed the RBT here, but it is important to note that regardless of parental approval, posting pictures of clients on social media is still prohibited. They have the right to privacy, and it is our responsibility to uphold that.

CHALLENGE 3: An RBT at your company is posting pictures of wounds on social media. She wrote that a client gave her these "battle scars." She also showed many pictures of an inflamed bite mark and wrote, "Some kids just need more help and I don't mind bleeding for them." Then the post continues with how "kids with autism *are* aggressive, but I was chosen for this job." She ends with a post using the client's initials with a plus sign next to hers.

RBT RESPONSE: You choose to comment under her post (on her Facebook page) about how unethical she is for posting about her client and providing misleading information about children with autism.

> *"Anyone can copy a photo and use it to make fun of or insult your client. Can you imagine how this will make the client or the family feel?"*

COMMENTARY: While the other RBT should not be posting about her clients or posting wrong information about autism, you should have either spoken to the RBT directly or told a supervisor. Commenting on her post is no better than if you made the original post yourself.

More Details

Posting a photo of a client on social media can have many dire, unintended consequences for the child.[4] First of all is the invasion of privacy that automatically occurs. Pictures on the internet are there in some form forever. A photo with a behavior analyst automatically designates the child as a client who needs services, most likely in some autism setting. What has to be taken into account is that the child will soon be an elementary and then a

4 https://jelliesapp.com/blog/5-reasons-not-to-post-about-your-child-on-social-media

middle-school student. The embarrassment they will feel if it is revealed that they were once labeled "autistic" could be devastating to them. Second, as an RBT, you should be concerned about the potential for your child client to be bullied by peers as they grow older. Anyone can copy a photo and use it to make fun of or insult your client. Can you imagine how this will make the client or the family feel? The internet allows anonymous comments by people who seem to enjoy harming or striking fear into others. Do you really want to subject your client to this form of bullying? Finally, all RBTs should be aware of "digital kidnapping" that now occurs on social media. This is a form of identity theft where someone takes a photo and uses it for their own twisted purposes. "Baby role-playing" involves someone who posts stolen pictures and then invents fake information about the child. They may create comments from the child's point of view that are disturbing and can even be malicious. In many cases, these kidnapped photos are used by people with mental health issues who want to be parents. Posting photos on social media or the internet gives license to anyone who wants to use the photos for sick purposes or fantasies.

Code 2.05 Test Yourself: Multiple-Choice

1. The agency you work for often posts on social media about their therapists and the company. Lately you have noticed they are posting pictures with children, and there was even a picture of one of *your* clients. The clients' names are never used, but you have recognized a few clients now. How should you respond?
   a. Go to your supervisor because you know it's unethical to be posting pictures of clients. Maybe the social media person doesn't know that.
   b. Just ignore the posts since you aren't responsible and didn't post these. Maybe they had the parents' permission.
   c. Comment on the post and say that the company is being unethical for posting pictures of clients.

   d. "Like" the post because you love your job and where you work and want to be supportive.
2. While scrolling through Instagram, you notice another RBT posted a picture of herself with a client and his family. How should you respond?
   a. Do nothing; it is unclear whether a violation has occurred.
   b. Assume that the parents provided consent, as they are in the picture; therefore, there is no violation.
   c. Ask if the parents gave consent. If they did, then no violation has occurred. If not, inform her that she is violating 2.05.
   d. Inform the RBT that she is violating 2.05. It doesn't matter if the parents gave consent.

Code 2.05 Test Yourself: True or False Questions

3. Another RBT from your company is posting about the BACB and how to obtain the RBT credential. This RBT only mentions the BACB and how to obtain credentials. This is ethical.

   True or False?

   True

   False
4. One of your clients loves playing with the face filters on Snapchat, so you let him use your phone as reinforcement. After getting your phone back, you see a response from one of your friends who wrote, "Aw, what a cutie! Who is that boy?" You quickly realize that this young man managed to send snaps to several of your friends. Letting him play with your phone in this way was a violation of Code 2.05.

   True or False?

   True

   False

For correct answers, go to Appendix A

2.06 RBTs ALWAYS OBTAIN PERMISSION FROM CLIENTS AND STAFF TO RECORD INTERVIEWS AND SERVICE DELIVERY SESSIONS. CONSENT MUST BE SPECIFICALLY AND SEPARATELY OBTAINED FROM EACH INDIVIDUAL

Quick Take

> "When it comes to human services, privacy and confidentiality are essential to the professional relationship and the general rule is 'No Recording'."

With video and audio recording apps on every phone, there is a temptation to record remarkable or fascinating events, from rock concerts to private conversations, for later analysis or evaluation. After all, you never know when you might need to review what transpired to entertain your friends or just to prove that you were right in your prediction of who would win the big game on Saturday. However, when it comes to human services, privacy and confidentiality are essential to the professional relationship, and the general rule is "No Recording." If you have been asked by your supervisor to record an interaction with the family or one of your therapy sessions, remember you must have written consent from anyone who is to appear on the recording. Your agency should have a consent form for just this purpose. Once signed, multiple copies should be distributed to all the parties, including the person giving the permission, yourself, and your supervisor. The consent form should include the date; time; location; purpose of the recording; and signature lines for the person(s) being recorded, yourself, and your supervisor. Note that this consent is a one off; that is, it can only be issued for one event, not a blanket consent for any extended period of time.

CHALLENGE 1: When you started having trouble making progress with a new client who engages in elopement, you asked your BCBA for more feedback and supervision time. Your supervisor told you that she does not have time right now to provide you with more supervision. She asked you to record your session and send it to her, and she said will watch it later and then give you feedback on your session.

RBT RESPONSE: You record your next session on your phone and send it to your supervisor as instructed.

COMMENTARY: Even though your supervisor asked you to send her the video, you still didn't have parental consent to record the session. Your supervisor should be making time to supervise you and shouldn't ask you to violate the code. As the RBT, you should remind your supervisor that recording the client without parental consent is not allowed under the RBT Code.

CHALLENGE 2: The behavioral team has reported having frequent issues during DTT with a particular client. Specifically, they often have difficulties completing trials due to low motivation and increased problem behaviors.

RBT RESPONSE: During one of your sessions, you identified a great reinforcer and made a video of the session so you can show the rest of the team.

COMMENTARY: Unless the RBT obtains written parental consent, this would be in violation. Before acting in a situation like this, it is always best to do some research. You are not allowed to record videos of clients without written parent consent.

"In some states, recording without permission is a third-degree felony punishable by fines and jail time."

More Details

Although the laws vary from one state to the next about recording a conversation, the RBT Ethics Code takes precedent. In our profession, the personal relationship between therapist/technician and our clients is always the most important. To be invited into a client's home or a teacher's classroom is a privilege and an honor to be respected, and a specially designated clinic is equally sacrosanct. The client deserves our respect and understands that theirs is a vulnerable situation where an audio or video clip could be taken out of context and ruin a relationship or someone's life. In each of these situations, the home, the classroom, or the clinic, the parents or teachers have a reasonable expectation of privacy, and if you were to make an audio or video recording that came to light, you could be arrested. In some states, recording without permission is a third-degree felony punishable by fines and jail time.

Code 2.06 Test Yourself: Multiple-Choice Questions

1. A client who is new to your program engages in high levels of problem behavior. This client's reduction-behavior protocol is complicated, and the other therapists have had issues implementing it. One of the other RBTs on this case asks you to record yourself implementing the protocol and send it to the other therapists as an example. How should you respond?
   a. I can totally do that; I am a team player.
   b. No; if you can't figure out how to implement the protocol, you should ask someone else.
   c. I would love to help, but it would be unethical to record the client without permission. We should talk to the supervisor about the protocol.
   d. Tell the other therapists yes but not actually record and say you forgot.
2. Parents have given consent to record part of your session with their child in school. You plan to record him and his teacher working 1:1. How should you proceed?
   a. You're all set to begin recording.

b. You must first obtain consent from the teacher, as she will be in the video.
c. Do not record; it is unethical to do so even if consent was obtained.
d. You can make an audio recording, but video recording is not permitted.

Code 2.06 Test Yourself: True or False Questions

3. Having obtained all the necessary parental consent to record a therapy session with a client, you decide to record a group of clients interacting and having fun with your client. This is appropriate because they all have social skills goals. This is allowed under the Code.

   True or False?

   True

   False

For correct answers, go toAppendix A

FOR FURTHER READING

Plunkett, L. A. (2019). *Sharenthood: Why We Should Think Before We Talk About Our Kids Online*. Boston: MIT Press.

www.care.com/c/stories/4275/5-dangers-of-social-media-to-discuss-with-you/

2.07 RBTs PROTECT THE CONFIDENTIALITY AND PRIVACY OF THEIR CLIENTS. RBTs ONLY USE RELEVANT IDENTIFYING INFORMATION IN THEIR JOB-RELATED COMMUNICATIONS (E.G., CONSULTATION, EMAILS, REPORTS). CONFIDENTIALITY AND PRIVACY REQUIREMENTS MAY BE ESTABLISHED BY LAW OR BY AN ORGANIZATION'S POLICIES

Quick Take

Section 2.07 of the Code addresses confidentiality and privacy. There are some differences between these two important concepts.

Confidentiality basically places restrictions on access to or releasing of certain types of information. There are legal protections in many professions related to confidentiality. An example is physician-patient privilege, which means doctors may not release records or reveal discussions with patients without their written permission. *Privacy* generally refers to respecting the boundaries related to someone's information of a personal or sensitive nature.

"The essence of Code item 2.07 is that information you gain about a client while you are on the job as an RBT may not be shared with others without the written consent of the person; that is, the information is confidential."

The essence of Code item 2.07 is that information you gain about a client while you are on the job as an RBT may not be shared with others without the written consent of the person; that is, the information is *confidential.* This is most likely to apply when you are working in a client's home. You are entitled to ask questions about how your client is doing in a general sense, and, more specifically, you may ask about the frequency of certain behaviors, antecedents that may have occasioned the behaviors, or consequences that followed. This is all part of your job as an RBT and is considered confidential in much the same way that a client reveals information in confidence to their lawyer (attorney-client privilege).

You would be *violating your client's privacy* if you began asking questions unrelated to your behavior analysis work, "So, how long have you been married?", "Do you plan to have other children?", "That's an interesting job you have. I'm just curious: how much do you make a year in take-home pay?" and, "Do you have plans for a Christmas vacation trip this year?" These would all be serious intrusions into the family's privacy, and asking such questions would be a violation of Code 2.07.

Advice to RBTs: The simplest rule to remember from 2.07 is *Don't Be Nosy*; just mind your own business. When you are preparing reports or memos about your behavior analytic work in the home, you may only include information that is relevant and obtained appropriately as part of your job. You may not release this information or talk about the client or client's family to anyone other than another direct service provider (e.g., "Jason's mother is in the hospital, so there will be a two-week lapse in services"). Your company should have specific guidelines for you to follow with regard to confidentiality and preparing/storing reports, data, and other written information. Finally, any information you may have overheard in conversations in a client's home is strictly off limits in reports or emails.

CHALLENGE 1: While you are working with your client in the classroom, the other students have started asking you why you are only helping Andrew.

RBT RESPONSE: You tell the students that Andrew has something called autism and sometimes he needs more help than others. You say that you are only there to help him learn to be like everyone else.

COMMENTARY: Sometimes it best to say that you are just there to help out and move on.

It is quite common for other students in your client's classroom to be interested in you. You are someone new in their classroom, and they see you playing and having fun with your client. Be prepared for these kinds of questions and have a statement ready to tell the other children when they ask what you are doing with your client. "I am just here to help out in the classroom" is always a good response; otherwise, you risk violating your client's confidentiality by telling the other students who you are and revealing confidential information, like a diagnosis, about your client.

CHALLENGE 2: At a team meeting for one of your clients, the other RBTs started talking about how "weird" the client's mom has been and that she has seemed "crazy." They also mentioned that the client's dad has not been present for any of the home sessions lately. After the last home session, mom explained that they are getting a divorce and dad is moving out, and she asked you not to tell anyone. The other RBTs asked you if you have heard anything.

RBT RESPONSE: "Oh, well, I do have something on that for you, but this is strictly hush-hush; apparently they are getting divorced, and dad is in the process of moving out. Mom didn't exactly say why, but I could tell by the anguish in her voice that dad must be cheating on her."

COMMENTARY: Not only did you violate the mother's *privacy*, you also presented the information as gossip and extrapolated on the information that the mother told you. If you felt like the events at home were affecting the client's behaviors, then the only person you should tell is your supervisor. It violates Code 2.07 by breaking the privacy of the client's mother to relay information that you did not have a right to.

CHALLENGE 3: A woman approached you while you were working with your client at the gym. She noticed your company shirt that is branded with their logo *Autism Treatment Specialists* and said that what you are doing is wonderful. She asked you how long you have worked with people with autism.

RBT RESPONSE: You politely tell the woman that you cannot talk right now and quickly direct your attention away from her.

COMMENTARY: Situations like this are uncomfortable and can be minimized by avoiding any clothing item that signals who you are and what you do.

"An RBT may only provide client information to someone other than the client 'for reasons of public interest'."

Although you did not technically breach *confidentiality*, your company's logo did. You and your company should work on modifying the current company shirt or policies associated with community sessions.

More Details

Like all health professionals, behavior analysts have a strict ethical and legal duty to keep client information confidential. Violating this duty could result in the RBT being disciplined by the BACB. In addition, the client could sue for breach of confidentiality. Note that an RBT may only provide client information to someone other than the client "for reasons of public interest."[5] This includes an illegal act of some kind, something dangerous to the public or to the client or her family, or in the case of some sort of emergency.

In the United States, based on the Constitution and common law, there is an assumed "right to privacy" that has existed since 1890. The general concept is that individual citizens have a basic "right to be left alone."[6]

Code 2.07 Test Yourself: Multiple-Choice Questions

1. The other RBTs at your job were discussing a client and his parents. The client's mother has recently spoken of her history with mental health problems, and she has said that raising a son with autism is hard for her. The RBTs were discussing how they think the mother doesn't love her son and they don't understand why. They ask if you know anything about the mother. How should you respond?
   a. "I can tell you, but you can't tell anyone."
   b. "We should get back to work."
   c. "I don't like to gossip about anyone, especially our clients."

5 https://lawhandbook.sa.gov.au/ch29s03.php
6 https://en.wikipedia.org/wiki/Privacy_law

d. "It would be violating the client's right to privacy to talk about this."

2. On a community outing, you were teaching your client how to push the cart around the grocery store when one of your friends walked up and asked if this was one of your clients with autism. How should you respond?
   a. Say that you can't really talk because you are helping your friend grocery shop and you can catch up later.
   b. Tell her yes and then introduce your friend to your client since greeting people is a social skills goal.
   c. Your friend already knows that he has autism, so you can just answer, "Yes."
   d. Ignore your friend and pretend like you have no idea who she is. She'll get the message.

   COMMENTARY: If you are working in schools or in the community, it is quite common to see someone you know. As an RBT, you should be prepared with a statement to tell that friend or family member about what you are doing that does not violate Code 2.07. It is no one else's business why you are helping that person, and your statement should be as short and give as little information as possible.

Code 2.07 Test Yourself: True or False Questions

3. During an in-home session, you notice there are some bruises on your client's arms and neck. These appear to be fresh bruises you didn't see the day before. You're aware you are ethically bound to ensure the welfare of your client, but you also don't want to violate the family's privacy. You decide to ask the client's mother about the bruises and the events that might have caused them. This is a violation of the Code.

   True or False?

   True

   False

4. Because you will be seeing your client tomorrow, you decided to leave his program binder in your car. When you pick up your significant other from work, she sees the binder and starts reading. "This is really interesting, Savannah," she says. You did not protect your client's confidentiality by leaving the binder where someone could see it.
   True or False?
   True
   False

For correct answers, go to Appendix A

2.08 RBTs ONLY DISCUSS CONFIDENTIAL INFORMATION WITH THOSE WHO NEED TO KNOW THAT INFORMATION. THEY SHARE INFORMATION FOR JOB-RELATED PURPOSES ONLY. CONFIDENTIAL INFORMATION INCLUDES, BUT IS NOT LIMITED TO: (1) INFORMATION ABOUT ANYONE WITH WHOM THE RBT WORKS; OR (2) INFORMATION ABOUT ANYONE TO WHOM THE RBT PROVIDES SERVICES. RBTs MAINTAIN CONFIDENTIALITY WHEN HANDLING RECORDS UNDER THEIR CONTROL. THIS INCLUDES RECORDS THAT ARE WRITTEN, ELECTRONIC, OR IN ANY OTHER FORMAT. HANDLING A RECORD MAY INCLUDE CREATION, STORAGE, ACCESS, TRANSFER, OR DISPOSAL

This Code item is closely related to 2.07. In this element, emphasis is placed on whom you may share "job-related" *confidential* information with, including people you work with, such as other RBTs and BCBA supervisors. This also includes the family of the client you are serving. This means you cannot talk with your family, roommate, or significant other about your clients, and you cannot share information about your clients with any other clients. As in Code 2.07, you must be very careful when handling sensitive client records or documents. This includes both hard copies or electronic versions, so that confidential information does not leak out to anyone who is not authorized to see the material. This is no easy task. You may be asked about your clients most any time of the day from people you run into at work or in the community, so you need your guard up. A casual conversation with the secretary at the front desk could be a test for you if he says, "So how is it going with Rebecca? I heard she had a meltdown yesterday." People will also ask about your clients when you are in the community. Someone in line behind you at the grocery store might say something like, "Hi, I recognize you. You work with my neighbor's daughter, don't you? She has autism. How is she doing?"

> *"This is no easy task; you may be asked about your clients most any time of the day from people you run into at work or in the community, so you need to keep your guard up."*

CHALLENGE 1: When you were in your favorite local taco shop, a former coworker came to your table and after a friendly greeting said, "How is Tyler doing? I miss him so much."

RBT RESPONSE: "Well, we finally got the head-banging under control, but now he's been doing a lot of biting. He's regressed on his potty training since you left, and he's having accidents all the time. His feeding program looks good, though; he's mastered bananas and carrots."

COMMENTARY: The RBT is in violation of 2.08. Regardless of the old coworker's past relationship to the client, she is no longer privy to this kind of information. When her professional relationship ended with the client, so did her access to client-related updates.

CHALLENGE 2: The parent of a client began asking questions about another child at your clinic. She says, "I don't understand why you guys are having Antonne ask for things that he wants, but you are having my Jayce use sign language. Antonne and Jayce are a lot alike, so why would it be different?"

RBT RESPONSE: "Well, right now we are really focusing on sign language with Jayce because sometimes when he gets upset, it is difficult to have him repeat a word. We can prompt him to sign for things, which allows useful communication. We are also still working on building his verbal imitation skills, which will help us to be able to build his verbal communication."

MOTHER RESPONSE: "But doesn't Antonne have problem behaviors, too? I always see him having tantrums in the waiting room. How is that different?"

RBT RESPONSE: "You know, I really can't talk about another client's treatment, but I can talk to my supervisor about setting up a meeting to discuss Jayce's program with you in more detail."

COMMENTARY: This RBT did a great job of redirecting the conversation away from discussing confidential information about another client, even when the mother continued to inquire. Some parents may choose to discuss this information with other parents, but that still does not allow you to provide this information.

CHALLENGE 3: One of your more difficult clients, Terrance, engages in severe aggression and has injured therapists to the point of causing bruising and bleeding. Another RBT from the clinic who does not work with Terrance came to you and initiated a conversation about him.

RBT 1: "Hey, I see you have another wound to add to your collection."

RBT 2: "Yeah, it hurts more than it looks like."

RBT 1: "How is it going with Terrance? I heard his aggression is getting worse every day. It doesn't seem like he has much of an aggression protocol."

RBT 2: "No, he really doesn't. We are told to block his attempts, and if he actually aggresses, then it was our fault for not blocking correctly. I don't think his lead therapist knows what she is doing."

> *"There can be penalties for breach of confidentiality, which may include termination of employment, as well as a possible civil suit or even criminal charges for violation of confidentiality."*

COMMENTARY: So, while it might be frustrating to work with a client that engages in severe aggression and to have a supervisor that doesn't seem to be helping, it is unethical to speak about the client and the client's protocols with an RBT that is not on the case. This information is confidential to those who work with the client. A better solution to your frustration would be to talk with the other RBTs on the client's case and then the supervisor.

More Details

When you joined your company, you probably signed an employment contract that very likely included a confidentiality agreement. Otherwise, confidentiality is implicit, except that it is included in the RBT Ethics Code, which makes it unethical to disclose such information. There can be penalties for breach of confidentiality, which may include termination of employment, as well as a possible civil suit or even criminal charges for violation of confidentiality. Finally, of course, you could be reported to the Board for violating the RBT Ethics Code and could be decertified.

Given all the possible severe negative outcomes from revealing confidential information, it is very clear that we take your handling of client information seriously and that having access to this information is a major ethical responsibility not to be taken lightly.

Code 2.08 Test Yourself: Multiple-Choice

1. While having lunch with a friend, she started asking about your job. She thinks she is interested in becoming an RBT, and she wanted to know about the clients and what you actually do during a day. How should you respond?
   a. "I can tell you about ABA and the types of clients we work with at my agency, but it would be unethical for me to discuss any of my actual clients with you."
   b. "It's the best job in the world, and you can basically set how many hours you want to work."
   c. "I'm not sure you would like it. I've been kicked, bitten, and scratched, and I sometimes work on weekends."
   d. "Well, I work with a bunch of different clients. Let me tell you about my favorite client, Marquis."
2. Many parents at your agency get together for coffee and to discuss their children and what they have learned about having a child with autism. They basically try to help any new parents that come along. When your client's mother came to pick her up, another parent was waiting on his child. The other parent stopped you and asked, "How is little Nia doing? Her mom said at our weekly coffee that her tantrums are getting worse." How should you respond?
   a. "Well, actually, the tantrums are getting worse, but it's because we started something new with her this week."
   b. "That's really nice of you to ask, but, as I'm sure you know, I can't discuss clients with other people. That would be unethical."
   c. "I'm not sure about her tantrums. If you really want to know, then ask Nia's mom."
   d. "UGH, YES. Her tantrums are worse, and it's getting really annoying."

3. The principal at the school where you are working pulled you aside and asked about a client's aggressive behaviors and how you are treating them. How should you respond?
   a. Provide all the information you have, as the principal is in a position of authority, and she has the right to know.
   b. You should not provide any information regarding the client's behaviors to anyone not involved in the treatment.
   c. Provide only information about the client's behavior plan, but do not provide any confidential information about the family, and so on.
   d. Refer the principal to your supervisor.

Code 2.08 Test Yourself: True False Questions

4. Under Code 2.08: Another RBT is asking questions about a client that you both work with in the school. She tells you that she has been struggling with his BIP (Behavior Intervention Plan) and would like to ask you some questions. You should not relay this information to her, as it would violate the client's confidentiality.

   True or False?
   True
   False

2.09 RBTs NEVER DISCLOSE CONFIDENTIAL INFORMATION WITHOUT CONSENT FROM THE CLIENT. EXCEPTIONS ARE MADE AS REQUIRED BY LAW, OR WHERE ALLOWED BY LAW FOR A VALID REASON. THIS INCLUDES, BUT IS NOT LIMITED TO: (1) PROVIDING NEEDED SERVICES; (2) OBTAINING APPROPRIATE CONSULTATIONS; AND (3) PROTECTING THE CLIENT OR OTHERS FROM HARM

Quick Take

This Code element is directly related to Codes 2.07 and 2.08 regarding confidentiality of client information. This is an essential

"If a sheriff's deputy contacts you regarding your client, they no doubt have a valid reason for making an inquiry, and sharing confidential information with them is permitted."

element of a trust relationship that we are trying to build with clients. The "consent from the client" phrase actually means *written* consent and is rarely given by the client unless there is some strong motivation to do so. If the family relies on an aunt, cousin, or neighbor for occasional respite care, the family may sign a consent form for these caregivers to be informed about the treatment plan. If the parents have contracted with an Occupational Therapist (OT) or Physical Therapist (PT) for services, you could safely assume that you could share information with them. Likewise, if a sheriff's deputy contacts you regarding your client, they no doubt have a valid reason for making an inquiry, and sharing confidential information with them is permitted.

CHALLENGE 1: When the treatment team was discussing a school-aged client in a meeting, the speech therapist said, "I've been trying to work on communication for a while now using a PECS book, but he hasn't made any progress. I don't really know what to do."

RBT RESPONSE: "We are using sign language instead of PECS because his visual discrimination skills are limited. We tried both PECS and sign language, and he has been doing so much better with sign language."

COMMENTARY: This would not be in violation, as the information is being provided to a speech therapist who has been contracted for services with this client.

CHALLENGE 2: Sign language is your client's primary form of communication. You have sent several signs on flash cards to the client's parents so they can use them when communicating with the client, Caden. You rarely see Caden's parents at the clinic. His grandmother always picks him up from sessions and allows you to have home sessions at her house. She has asked for a list of Caden's signs so she can communicate with him, but the client's mother has told your supervisor not to give any information to grandma. You assume there is a personal issue between them.

RBT RESPONSE: You decide that grandma deserves to know what is going on with her grandson, and you think it's awesome that she wants to know his signs so she can talk to him. You feel that grandma is more invested in the therapy than the parents, and it's not fair that she isn't allowed to know, so you print off the sign language cards and give them to her at the next session.

COMMENTARY: Even though you are an RBT and are providing therapy to the child, you are really working with the entire family. It might seem unfair that the grandmother isn't allowed to have any information regarding her grandson despite how involved she appears to be, but the mother has requested that she doesn't want any information given to the grandmother. Basically, it would be unethical for you to discuss anything with grandmother and a breach of confidentiality in this situation.

> *"This historic commitment to confidentiality is deep and binding for a good reason."*

More Details

The basic principle of confidentiality goes all the way back to the Hippocratic Oath from the 10th century. By way of our RBT Ethics Code, the Oath is extended to our behavioral profession. This historic commitment to confidentiality is deep and binding for a good reason. Professionals who work closely with clients as we do need to be aware of private information that could be very relevant to our understanding of the client's behavior, the history behind certain response patterns, or motivational variables associated with performance over time. If this information were to leak out, it could be very embarrassing to the family or even lead to tragic consequences. If the client had a history of making threatening comments such as, "I'm going to kill myself," you would want the parents to tell you so that your ABA team could build in the necessary protections when they are working with the client, as well as seeking appropriate input from other professionals.

Code 2.09 Test Yourself: Multiple-Choice Questions

1. The OTs have asked for RBTs to be present at OT sessions due to the client's severe aggression. The OTs have also asked the RBTs to help intervene during times of problem behavior. In an OT session, the OT asked what goals you are currently working on with the client. How should you respond?
   a. "Why do you want to know about behavior goals? Are you going to use these also?
   b. "Well, we are mostly working on communication skills right now, so the aggression should start to decrease."
   c. "I'm sorry, I can't share that information since you aren't an RBT."
   d. "I don't know. My supervisor doesn't tell me anything."
2. Dalia, a school-aged student (and your client), lives with her mother due to a divorce agreement. Your supervisor informed you that Dalia's mother has custody and should be the only parent to receive treatment updates about Dalia. As you are leaving your session, Dalia's dad stops you in the parking lot to ask you how she is doing. How should you respond?
   a. "Oh, I am so glad to see you! You are really the only parent who cares about Dalia's progress."

b. "I'm really sorry; I can't make any comment. Please feel free to contact my supervisor."
c. "I am sorry. I can't talk to you since Dalia's mother has custody."
d. "If you call me later, I can update you on the phone."

Code 2.09 Test Yourself: True False Questions

3. During a community session with your client at the mall, the client began to engage in an emotional outburst and started yelling, "Stranger Danger! I don't know her. Someone help me!" The mall police officer asked you for identification and your relationship to the child. You gave the officer your driver's license and agency ID and told the officer you are a behavior therapist there to help the child. You told him that he could contact the school or child's mother and gave him the contact information. Providing client information in this situation is a violation of the Code.

   True or False?
   True
   False
4. A substitute teacher was working in the classroom for the day. The substitute told you that the regular teacher informed her that you would be coming in to work with Hann. She asked why you were only helping your client and not the other students. You decided this teacher needed to know why you were there, so you told the substitute that your client has autism and you are a behavior therapist who is there to help him during the day. Explaining this is not an ethical violation.

   True or False?
   True
   False
5. At drop-off, a parent told you, "His uncle will be picking him up today. Feel free to give him a run-down of how the session went, and he will pass the information along

to me." When the uncle came to pick up the client, you made sure to give him a detailed overview of the treatment session. Giving the uncle the overview is a violation of Code 2.09.

True or False?
True
False

For correct answers, go toAppendix A

2.10 RBTs CREATE, MAINTAIN, DISTRIBUTE, STORE, RETAIN, AND DISPOSE OF RECORDS AND DATA RELATING TO THEIR SERVICES (1) IN ACCORDANCE WITH APPLICABLE LAWS, REGULATIONS, AND POLICIES; (2) IN A WAY THAT COMPLIES WITH THE REQUIREMENTS OF THIS CODE; AND (3) IN A MANNER THAT ALLOWS FOR APPROPRIATE TRANSITION OF SERVICE AT ANY GIVEN TIME

Quick Take

There is a lot of paperwork associated with the delivery of behavior analysis services. The documents' primary purpose is to record all aspects of the client's behavior from initial assessment to final discharge. Third-party payers (insurance, Medicare) require this documentation to verify that the service was delivered. As behavior analysts, we need all of this data to show progress in behavior change over time. As an RBT, you will be responsible for recording data, keeping the data sheets up to date, and graphing this data on a regular basis so that your behavior analysis team can analyze it and make changes in the

"As an RBT, you will be responsible for recording data, keeping the data sheets up to date, and graphing this data on a regular basis."

program if necessary. Many companies are moving to electronic data collection and automatic graphing, which can make all of this much easier to use and maintain. As the primary therapist, your job is to ensure the accurate recording of treatment data and pay close attention to the behavior plan to ensure treatment integrity. The maintenance, distribution, storage, retention, and disposal of these records will generally be done by your BCBA or someone else at your company.

A secondary purpose of all of this documentation is to allow a smooth transition to another therapist if you should leave the agency or possibly to another provider if the client is discharged.

CHALLENGE 1: Not quite caught up with technology, your agency is still using paper programs and data sheets. Your BCBA told you the programs that were handed out at the last meeting apparently did not print correctly and to use the new ones that were just dropped off. The next therapist just told you to throw away these programs since there isn't any data on them.

RBT RESPONSE: You decide that it's fine to toss the data sheets away since there isn't any data on them, and it's not like the teachers would understand what the programs mean anyway.

COMMENTARY: While it might seem harmless just to throw written behavior programs away, even if there isn't any data recorded and only client names and target behaviors are on there. You need to take the programs back to your clinic and shred them properly; otherwise, it is a code violation. Your company no doubt has a policy for disposing of behavior programs; they should never be thrown away in a place like a school.

CHALLENGE 2: With your agency specializing in community sessions (i.e. school, social group, home), it is customary to leave the client's written programs at the location where the program took place. For a while, you and the other therapists were leaving your client's programs in a locked cabinet in the classroom. Your client now starts his day in a different classroom, and you and the other therapists are tired of walking to the other side of the school for his programs.

RBT RESPONSE 1: "I am so tired of getting here ten minutes earlier than I need to, ten minutes I'm not being paid, just to pick up his programs. I found a really tall bookshelf in the new classroom. We could leave his programs on top of that, and no one but us will even know they are there."

RBT RESPONSE 2: "I know it's frustrating, but we should lock up his programs. It would be unethical for us to leave them out where anyone could find them. Leaving his programs on a bookshelf in public could breach his confidentiality and violate Code 2.10. We should ask the teacher if we can lock them in a drawer or cabinet."

COMMENTARY: RBT 2 handled this situation really well by adhering to code 2.10 but also presenting an idea of how to solve the frustration and extra effort of obtaining the programs.

> *"The documentation needs to be complete enough that a new behavior analysis treatment team can pick up right where yours left off. The goal is a seamless transition so that the client does not regress or lose valuable skills."*

More Details

It is not unusual for clients to move from one agency to another or for the family to relocate to another state. In this case, they will want a clear record of the assessment results and treatment outcomes that their child had, as well as the behavior intervention and support plans. The documentation needs to be complete enough that a new behavior analysis treatment team can pick up right where yours left off. The goal is a seamless transition so that the client does not regress or lose valuable skills. The data that needs to be kept does not include the raw data from daily data sheets as long as that data was converted to table or graphic form. The laws, regulations, and policies regarding the maintenance, distribution, storage, retention, and disposal of these records vary from one state to the next, so your clinical director will need to be in charge of all of these duties and obligations. Your primary job is to make sure that the data you have entered is correct, valid, and reliable per any integrity checks that need to be recorded.

Code 2.10 Test Yourself: True False Question

1. When you were with your client on the playground, you placed your clipboard containing the data sheet on the picnic table. You turned around and realized all the teachers had come over and taken seats at the table. They did not appear to have looked at your data sheet, but you decided it was best to quickly grab the data sheet and remove it from the table just in case. Leaving your clipboard on the table is not an ethical violation.

   True or False?
   Truc
   False

For correct answers, go toAppendix A

6

Section 3—Competence and Service Delivery Codes 3.01–3.08

Section 2 emphasized the need of RBTs to closely protect the rights of clients and their confidential information, as well as avoiding "gifting" and any forms of discrimination against clients or their families. In Section 3, the emphasis shifts to more operational aspects of the job of being an ethical RBT. Codes 3.01 and 3.02 relate to your relationship with your supervisor, which should be close and professional. Your supervisor will guide you through the maze of behavior-analytic procedures necessary to produce effective behavior change. Supervisors will expect RBTs to keep them informed of any problems that they might be having, especially if the problem involves giving an assignment that is out of the RBT's range of competence. Being able to say, "I don't feel comfortable with . . . " should be a staple of your interactions, as well as, "Could you teach me how to . . . " These close interactions are intended to give you competencies in a variety of areas, including but not limited to data collection, graphing data, conducting preference assessments, and assisting with functional assessment procedures (Code 3.03).

In addition to learning new methods and procedures, you may be introduced to unfamiliar client populations (Code 3.04), and you will need to have the necessary training and supervision to practice competently. Code 3.05 stresses the importance of providing behavioral services only when you are hired and supervised to do so.

As an RBT, you will be interacting most of the time with clients or citizens who have basically no knowledge of our field and our special, technical terminology, which is why we have Code 3.06. This code item reminds all behavior analysts that they need to speak in easy-to-understand ways that communicate exactly what they are doing and why. You should basically avoid jargon at all times, except when you are with other RBTs or behavior analysts in your clinic, agency, or company.

As you learned in your 40-hour RBT training, data collection is at the heart of ABA and the graphing of that data requires special attention to conventions adopted by researchers and clinicians alike. These conventions are displayed in Figure 6.1. Graphs of data are used to make important decisions about client treatment, so they need to be carefully prepared to allow efficient determinations of trends and outcomes of interventions.

As mentioned in Section 1, there are many, many questionable, even dangerous, products, dubious methods, and wild untested theories of treatment that exist in our culture. In many respects, our solid, some say "boring," evidence-based approach is in the minority when compared to the world of fantasy interventions. Parents, teachers, and even some other professionals get caught up in these unproven treatments. As an RBT in a home, school, or multi-modal clinic, you may be asked to assist in the delivery of these questionable treatments. If this were to occur, two things need to happen: 1) immediately inform your supervisor, and 2) make sure that your RBT credential is not paired with the problematic intervention.

3.01 RBTs ONLY PRACTICE UNDER THE CLOSE, ONGOING SUPERVISION OF A QUALIFIED SUPERVISOR

Quick Take

As an RBT, you are no doubt aware that you must operate under close, ongoing supervision and that your supervisor has to have been *approved* or "qualified" by the BACB to serve as a supervisor.

RBT supervisors must have the following qualifications: BCBA®, BCBA-D™, or BCaBA (effective November 2019), OR be an individual licensed in another behavioral health profession that has applied behavior analysis in its legislative scope of practice and who is competent in applied behavior analysis.[1] Before providing any supervision, RBT supervisors must complete training based on the 8-hour Supervision Training Curriculum Outline, and they must earn 3 hours of continuing education per 2-year cycle.[2]

We would define "close" supervision as your supervisor directly observing you as you work with clients, taking data on your performance, and meeting with you afterward to provide you with feedback and training that employs a Behavioral Skills Training model.

To find a potential qualified supervisor, one option is to look on the BACB's Registry of Certificants. Step 1: Go to BACB.com and click on "Find a Certificant," then click "Find a BCBA/BCaBA." Step 2: Type in your search criteria, such as the last name of your potential BCBA supervisor, and click on "SEARCH." Once you have found your potential supervisor, click on that person's name, and a screen will come up that gives you all of the information on the person's credentials, including the bottom line, where it says, "Supervision." Following this, it tells you if the BCBA meets the current supervision requirements and whether they have any sanctions against them.

CHALLENGE 1: Rachel, a BCBA, recently obtained her certification and was assigned to supervise you. You've previously worked as an RBT and have heard that the way

1 Note: These individuals may only supervise RBTs under the oversight of an RBT requirements coordinator who is employed at the same organization as the licensed professional.

2 For more information, see: www.bacb.com/wp-content/uploads/RBT-Supervision-and-Supervisor-Requirements_190529.pdf

Rachel is practicing does not exactly meet the standards. She often appears overwhelmed, has difficulty answering simple questions about client protocols, never models procedures when training, and gives no specific feedback. You are about to begin accruing hours for your BCaBA and do not feel confident that this supervisor will provide you with a comprehensive fieldwork experience.

RBT RESPONSE: You set up a meeting with the clinical director and say, "I'd like to discuss the possibility of being transferred to Nicole's team. I will begin accruing hours for my BCaBA soon and feel that her extensive experience will be very beneficial in my training."

COMMENTARY: If this RBT is not transferred to a more competent supervisor, she will probably be better suited leaving this company. As a supervisee pursuing certification, it is in your best interest to find a supervisor who will provide you with the highest-quality training.

CHALLENGE 2: It is time to renew your RBT certification. You need to sign the paperwork, but you mention to your supervisor that you haven't been supervised at least 5% of your hours by a qualified supervisor. Your supervisor tells you that she is well aware of your sessions. You know this isn't true, since you haven't seen her in a month, and you are actually supervised by another RBT. Your supervisor tells you to go ahead and sign the paperwork, and she will make sure that you make up the hours later in the month.

WHAT *NOT* TO DO: You sign the paperwork and submit your recertification. Your supervisor knows best, and she said she would make up the hours. If your paperwork is late, there is a fee, and you don't want to get in trouble.

WHAT *TO* DO: You decide to discuss with your supervisor your concerns regarding the lack of supervision and wait to sign off on the paperwork until the requirements have been met.

COMMENTARY: By signing the paperwork, you are attesting that the necessary supervision requirements have been met. Upholding these requirements is critical for the RBT, as noncompliance could result in termination of their certification or eligibility to recertify. Although the BACB allows for the responsible assessor (BCaBA, BCBA, or BCBA-D) to delegate assessment components to an assistant assessor (who may be an RBT), the 5% supervision is still required to be conducted by a responsible supervisor. If you are uncertain of how this is arranged at your company, you should request clarification to ensure you are in compliance with all current standards, including recent updates.

CHALLENGE 3: The director of your company just sent you an email that said the only BCBA is quitting. She goes on to say that they do not have a replacement but should have one "in a few weeks." The director goes on to say, "Just follow your current schedule until we find a new supervisor."

RBT RESPONSE: "Thank you for letting me know. Are you going to provide my supervision, since I can't provide services without a supervisor?"

DIRECTOR RESPONSE: "No, but you'll be fine, trust me."

COMMENTARY: When an RBT no longer has a BCBA supervisor, they need to immediately cease providing behavior analytic services. There are no exceptions.

> *"Supervision gonc wrong can be a nightmare: 'I haven't seen my supervisor in three months.'"*

More Details

Good supervision is the heartbeat of behavior analysis practice. When supervision is done correctly, the supervisor and RBT are working as a close-knit team, revising treatment methods based on reliable data, having intense discussions about where to go next with the treatment plan, and sharing the joys of clients meeting one goal after another. Supervision gone wrong can be a nightmare. "I haven't seen my supervisor in three months," is what one RBT wrote in to the *ABAEthicsHotline*. Another wrote, "My supervisor never gives me any feedback, she just says, 'You're doing fine,' when I know that I'm not." One thing all supervisees need to realize is that supervisors need reinforcement, too. A good supervisor (one that is observing you, shaping your behavior, etc.) needs to hear from their RBTs that their efforts are appreciated and that RBTs feel they are improving their skills *because* of their supervisor.

Ongoing supervision means that your supervisor is meeting the minimum 5% requirement with you, which, depending on how many hours you work, should be once per week or at least every other week. All of this should have been specified in your RBT Supervision Contract that you reviewed with your supervisor and you both signed (be sure to keep a copy of that contract). Not mentioned in this Code is that if for some reason your supervisor leaves the company and there is no one to fill the supervisor position, you are not able to continue working. Also not mentioned is that, as an RBT, you have to take some responsibility for requesting your observation/supervision sessions from one to the next. If you don't ensure the observation sessions are scheduled, there could be a lapse in your supervision, and you will be out of compliance with this Code item. It is also important to note that you also have to take some responsibility for having documentation for your supervision. The documentation that you should be maintaining includes:

- 40-hour training certificate.
- RBT Competency Assessment annually.
- Documentation that supervision was conducted in accordance with the RBT supervision requirements. These include:
    - Documentation that 5% of RBT behavior analytic service hours were supervised

- Two face-to-face meetings per month with the RBT supervisor
- At least one of the meetings is a one-on-one meeting.
- At least one of the meetings includes *direct observation* of the RBT working with a client.
- Annual renewal with signed attestation by RBT that supervision was in accordance with the BACB standards.

There is a sample RBT Supervision Log at: www.bacb.com/wp-content/uploads/RBT-Audit-Documentation-and-Supervision-Log-181227.pdf

Code 3.01 Test Yourself: Multiple-Choice Questions

1. Your company has undergone many changes within its structure, and you are now working under a different BCBA. You have been working with the same clients, but you haven't been supervised in a while. When you asked for more supervision, your supervisor told you that more supervision is on the way. At your next session, a senior-level RBT showed up and said she was there to supervise you. How should you respond?
   a. "Great you're here. Let me show you the problems I am having."
   b. "Well, I was really hoping for the BCBA. You're an experienced therapist, but you don't meet the requirements to be a *qualified* supervisor. I am going to follow up about the BCBA coming."
   c. "Please don't take this the wrong way, but I need a real supervisor."
   d. "Wait. You're on my level. According to the code, you can't train me."
2. As a part of some reorganization, several months ago, your supervisor assigned you to work in-home sessions with a client who lives far from the supervisor's home. The supervisor told you that she will try to make it out when she can but will not be able to come often. Four

months have gone by, and the supervisor still has not come to a session. You have talked about the client with the supervisor in the office but really need to be observed and receive more feedback. How should you respond?

a. Wait and see if the supervisor comes. In the event that 6 months have passed, and she still has not come, you will then need to take action.
b. Take better notes during your meetings to ensure you are following all of her recommendations with integrity.
c. Ask more detailed questions during your meetings to receive more accurate recommendations.
d. Ask to receive more direct observation and supervision and, if not obtained, request to be taken off of the case. Put this in writing.

Code 3.01 Test Yourself: True or False Questions

3. One of the RBTs at your company just received her master's in ABA and will be sitting for her exam in a few months. The director informed you that the RBT will now be your supervisor and you will be receiving supervision strictly from the RBT. This would *not* be a violation, as an RBT can assume the role of a responsible supervisor once a master's in ABA has been obtained.

   True or False?
   True
   False

4. Your supervisor will be going on maternity leave and has arranged for another BCBA at the company to take over her cases as well as supervision while she is gone. This is standard, ethical practice.

   True or False?
   True
   False

For correct answers, go to Appendix A

3.02 RBTs FOLLOW THE DIRECTION OF THEIR SUPERVISORS AND INFORM THEM WHEN THEY ARE ASKED TO DO SOMETHING THAT GOES BEYOND THE SCOPE OF THEIR CERTIFICATION

Quick Take

> *"It might sound exciting and challenging to develop a functional assessment for a client, but your Task List says that you only 'Assist with functional assessment procedures.'"*

As an RBT, your "scope" of practice is defined by the RBT Task List (2nd ed.). Your supervisor should not ask you to do anything beyond that list. If he does, you need to let him know that you are not allowed to exceed your scope of practice; in other words, *push back* in a polite but firm manner. It might sound exciting and challenging to *develop* a functional assessment for a client, but your Task List says that you only "*Assist* with functional assessment procedures." If your supervisor asked you to develop a functional assessment, you would need to remind him about this limitation. The same goes for preference assessments, skill acquisition plans, and task analyses. RBTs are only allowed to *conduct* and carry out these procedures rather than developing them. If you review the Task List, you will see the words "implement," "conduct," and "assist" used throughout, but the words "develop" or "create" are not used to describe your role as an RBT.

The way in which you handle a discussion with your supervisor if you have been asked to do something not on the RBT Task List is critical to your success as an RBT. You should not sound defiant or obstructive in informing your supervisor of the limits imposed by the Task List. "I would love to learn more about how a functional assessment is developed, and I am more than happy to participate in that assessment," is more acceptable than, "No, I'm not going to needs to start with small approximations, not the full word. It seems that you were so excited and honored that you jumped the gun and went beyond the scope of your training.

More Details

The RBT title was created as an entry-level position in the behavior analysis delivery system. BCBAs have advanced training in behavioral theory and applied research and are expected to *create* individualized assessments, task analyses, and functional assessment procedures, as well as designing contingency systems to motivate clients. BCBAs train their RBTs to carry out these tasks, as well as providing necessary support and regular supervision. The Task List says, "It is at the discretion of an RBT supervisor to determine any activities outside of this task list that a behavior technician is competent to perform as a behavior technician." However, it is still up to you to let your supervisor know if you have the skills necessary to complete an assigned task, especially if it is beyond the scope of your certification. An RBT operating outside their scope of practice can cause harm. This is why operating outside of the scope of practice is unethical.

Code 3.02 Test Yourself: Multiple-Choice Questions

1. As a senior-level RBT, you have been working at the same clinic for a few years. Your clinic just hired new behavior therapists who haven't taken their RBT test yet. Typically, it is the supervisors who conduct all the training for the new hires, but there were so many hires, the supervisor can't train them all. Your supervisor has decided to have you do the training. How should you respond?
   a. "This sounds like an interesting challenge."
   b. "Um, are you sure you want me training them? I don't think I'm that good."

   c. "I've never trained another therapist before and that seems out of my scope of practice."
   d. "Am I allowed to train other therapists?"
2. Having recently learned about the different types of preference assessments, you want to get some experience with them. Which of the following is an appropriate way to do this?
   a. Ask your supervisor about assisting with or observing during an upcoming preference assessment.
   b. Develop and implement a preference assessment for one of your clients you feel could use one. As long as you feel confident in how to implement it, you do not need to consult your supervisor.
   c. Do not develop a preference assessment on your own, as that would violate 3.02, but if you find a protocol that is already written, you can practice it on your clients without needing to consult the supervisor.
   d. As long as you gain your supervisor's approval, you can create and implement a preference assessment independently.

Code 3.02 Test Yourself: True or False Questions

3. Along with your supervisor, you are working on creating a preference assessment for a client. Your supervisor asks you to create a list of potential edible reinforcers since you are typically there with the client during lunchtime and have seen what the client eats. This meets the requirements of Code 3.02.

   True or False?
   True
   False
4. Because you have worked in the field for a number of years, your supervisor trusts you. He asked you to conduct an Assessment of Functional Living Skills (AFLS) assessment,

an activity beyond the RBT task list. You feel confident that you can figure out how to do this on your own, even if you do not have direct experience with AFLS. You tell the supervisor you will do this. This is perfectly acceptable.

True or False?

True

False

5. As a fairly new RBT, you have only entered data and updated graphs for a few clients. This is a task that is listed on the RBT task list, and your supervisor has asked you to do this for a client. You do not really feel confident that you can complete this task correctly on your own, but you say that you will do the assignment because it is something you are supposed to know how to do. You're going to just give it your best shot. This violates 3.02.

   True or False?

   True

   False

For correct answers, go to Appendix A

3.03 RBTs MUST BE COMPETENT IN THE AREAS IN WHICH THEY PROVIDE BEHAVIOR TECHNICIAN SERVICES

> *"It is expected that you will perform to the best of your ability with a high level of proficiency."*

Quick Take

Your scope of practice was outlined in Code 3.02 and detailed in the RBT Task List. In Code 3.03, the discussion turns to your "competence" in providing those services. It is expected that you will perform to the best of your ability with a high level of proficiency. Your supervisor will determine your skill level when he administers the RBT Renewal Competency Assessment

Packet annually, but your regular supervision sessions serve the same function in real time every week. It is expected that you will be knowledgeable and experienced in four major areas: Measurement, Assessment, Skill Acquisition and Behavior Reduction, and Professionalism. For each of these, you will need to demonstrate your skill (e.g., using a partial-interval measurement system) or describe in an interview how you would handle a situation (e.g., maintaining professional boundaries). If you do this successfully and demonstrate mastery of the skill or concept, then you will have met the competence criterion.

CHALLENGE 1: An RBT colleague you were observing asked a client who was having an emotional outburst to explain what she was feeling. The RBT asked the client, Elena, what made her upset, and how she was feeling about completing her homework. After the session, you asked the RBT what program she was doing when Elena began to engage in the emotional outburst.

RBT 1 RESPONSE: "Oh, I wasn't running a specific program; I just wanted Elena to know that she was safe and could talk about what was upsetting her."

RBT 2 RESPONSE: "Oh, well, the thing is, you gave a lot of attention to the tantrum when the protocol says to ignore the outburst and keep prompting her to complete her work."

RBT 1 RESPONSE: "Yes, but I was asking about her feelings because I don't really know what else we are supposed to do when she has an outburst; this is what I learned in my undergraduate counseling class.

RBT 2 RESPONSE: "If you are confused on how to implement the reduction behavior protocol, I'm sure our supervisor would be happy to give you more training.

RBT 1 RESPONSE: "Okay, but I just don't want to look stupid."

COMMENTARY: RBT 2 was right to ask about the "counseling" procedures being implemented by RBT 1, who also seems to need training on identifying possible antecedents for Elena's outbursts.

CHALLENGE 2: The company where you have recently become employed has assigned you to a case involving an intensive feeding program. You mentioned in your interview that you had "some experience" in this area. In reality, you worked briefly on a case that involved mild food avoidance behaviors. The supervisor sent you the protocol and said, "Here is all of the information. We are just using escape extinction, so it's pretty straight forward. With your feeding experience, it should be no problem."

RBT RESPONSE: "I'm sorry; I've actually never implemented escape extinction with a feeding program. I will need some training and supervision. Are there any sessions that I can observe so I can get a better idea of what it looks like?"

COMMENTARY: This RBT certainly should not have implied she had more experience on a complex treatment such as feeding, but she did the right thing by confessing before this became a potentially dangerous situation.

CHALLENGE 3: Along with several other RBTs, you are working with a new client who engages in severe aggression. Another RBT, Sharon, who is also assigned to the client, told you that she has never worked with aggression, and she doesn't really know what to do. The BCaBA who trained Sharon gives her different reduction behavior protocols every week, and no one seems to know how to handle the aggression. Sharon told you that she doesn't know how much longer she can work with this client.

RBT RESPONSE: Following this session, you tell your supervisor that you don't feel comfortable working with this client. You tell your supervisor that you would first like experience working with a less severe behavior problem.

COMMENTARY: This is a classic example of an RBT just being thrown onto a case without proper supervision and training. It is quite common for an RBT to be added to a new case because there is a desperate need for more therapists or there are only a few therapists who are approved with a certain insurance company. No matter what behaviors the client engages in, as the RBT, you need to be competent in that area in order to provide services. Unfortunately, in this case, more than one RBT is involved.

"An RBT who is expert at prompting and fading techniques can subtly move a client toward a new food that was previously rejected or toward a highly rewarding play experience with peers."

More Details

The emphasis on competence could not be more important. How behavioral services are delivered means the difference between a client learning a critical skill at just the right time vs. missing an opportunity to come into contact with a pivotal experience that could open new doors. An RBT who is expert at prompting and fading techniques can subtly move a client toward a new food that was previously rejected or toward a highly rewarding play experience with peers. On the other hand, the incompetent application of DRO (Differential Reinforcement of Other behavior) (e.g., occasionally, accidentally, and reinforcing the target behavior) could lead to prolonged tantrums that interrupt overall progress toward larger socialization goals. Precision in timing the delivery of reinforcers or adjusting the requirements for a reward in shaping a chain of behavior is critical to the administration of behavior analytic services. *Competence is what we do; it's who we are.* The short-term and long-term harm to clients from services delivered by an incompetent RBT is what makes a situation unethical.

Code 3.03 Test Yourself: Multiple-Choice Questions

1. While you are working on a program that involves a DRO procedure, one day you arrive early for your session and notice that another tech is running the program differently than you are. When you show her how you have been doing it, she says you are actually implementing non-contingent reinforcement (NCR). What should you do?
   a. Continue running the program as you have been and wait to see if your supervisor corrects you.
   b. Assume that the other technician is right and begin implementing it the way she did.
   c. Ask your supervisor if she can clarify the differences between DRO and NCR and practice implementing them with you.
   d. First try to work it out on your own. If you admit to your supervisor that you are not competent, she will most likely have you take your RBT renewal early.

Code 3.03 Test Yourself: True or False Questions

2. Another RBT was conducting a session with a client as you observed. The client frequently engages in multiple forms of stereotypy when expected to be on task. You noticed that the RBT was reinforcing the stereotypy by calling it "cute" and telling the client that he doesn't have to work. When you asked the RBT about reinforcing the stereotypy, she said, "Well, it's not really a problem behavior, so what's the issue with reinforcing it?" This attitude is unethical.

   True or False?

   True

   False
3. When your supervisor conducted your RBT renewal assessment, she only asked you to describe the common functions of behavior but did not directly test you on your assessment *in vivo*. This approach is a violation of 3.03.

True or False?
True
False

4. You recently completed the RBT Renewal Competency Assessment, during which your supervisor just checked off all the areas without direct testing. She said, "I know you can do all of this, so there is no use in doing it again." You are feeling a little uneasy because there are some areas for which you don't have the skills, but you just go along with it anyway. This is a violation of 3.03.

True or False?
True
False

For correct answers, go to Appendix A

3.04 RBTs MAY NOT PRACTICE WITH NEW CLIENT POPULATIONS WITHOUT PROPER TRAINING AND OVERSIGHT

Quick Take

> *"What you are looking for is a location where you can apply what you know already about behavior analysis and receive on-the-job training under a new supervisor who has expertise in this area."*

In your first job as an RBT, you will be working with some specific populations, such as children diagnosed with Autism Spectrum Disorder. Your work might be done at a clinic or in a public school, and your new supervisor will train you and ease you into your job, Hopefully, you will immediately begin to pick up skills and gain confidence. As you become proficient with this population, you may be exposed to other types of clients, such as delinquent youths or adults with developmental disabilities, and you might decide that you would like to try working with them next. So, what do you do? You could start looking for jobs online where they are hiring RBTs and set up some interviews, but what if they ask you what expertise you have in this area? You could fake it and lead them to believe that you have experience, but that would be unethical. The right approach is to ask your supervisor if the company has other branches where different populations receive treatment. Ask if you can visit as an observer (on your own time). This will also give you a chance to talk to the RBTs who work there and ask questions about how they got trained. You can also ask for tips on how to get a job there. If you believe that this type of setting is for you, it is time to start learning as much as you can about that population by reading, going to conferences, and attending workshops. In a few months, you should have a good grasp of what it will take to make the move, and you can start looking for a job with that population. What you are looking for is a location where you can apply what you know already about behavior analysis and receive on-the-job training under a new supervisor who has expertise in this area. This is the ethical way to learn treatment methods and procedures for a new population.

CHALLENGE 1: You have primarily treated early intervention clients with ASD at the company where you are working. Your supervisor informed you of a new ASD client you will be assigned to who is 18 years old. The supervisor said that this case will focus on higher-level social skills training and facilitating independence at the client's job. As it turns out, you have no experience in either of these areas.

RBT RESPONSE: "Wow that sounds great! I am excited to get some experience with a different population. Do you recommend any good articles that will help me get up to speed? Can you tell me a little bit about the older clients you've worked with to give me a better idea of what his treatment will look like?"

COMMENTARY: A message like this might help serve as a subtle prompt to the supervisor, reminding her of your lack of experience. This also allows you to gauge your supervisor's expertise in this area to ensure she has the necessary experience to train you to competency.

CHALLENGE 2: The new town where you just moved is relatively smaller than the mid-sized city you just left. You are busy looking for your next job. There are only a few ABA clinics in this new town, and only one invited you for an interview after you sent out your résumé to them all. This clinic only works with people who have dementia and live in assisted living homes. When you went for your interview, the BCBA asked you how long you have worked with adults who have dementia.

WHAT NOT TO DO: You really need this job and none of the other agencies are currently hiring, so you tell the BCBA that you have the experience and loved working with this population.

WHAT *TO* DO: Although you are concerned you may not get a job offer, you decide it would be best to be honest. You let the BCBA know that although you do not have any experience with this population, you are very interested in learning more, are a quick study, and would appreciate the opportunity to receive training.

COMMENTARY: Even though it might seem difficult to move somewhere new and have to look for a job, it is unethical to say you are competent working

"Once you feel you are prepared to leave your current job, you will need to give them adequate notice so they can find your replacement. Otherwise, your clients may not receive the treatment that they expect."

with a population with which you have no experience. It's possible that this BCBA would be open to training you to work with this population, but you should not be practicing without the necessary training.

More Details

Transitioning to a new population presents several ethical challenges. First, you will need to be honest with your current supervisor about your interest in changing positions and ask for her assistance in learning about this category of individuals. Next, you will need to arrange to visit settings where these people receive treatment, and you will have to be screened and background-checked, just like your first job. You will also have to sign a confidentiality agreement since you may be exposed to confidential information about the clients in this setting. And, finally, once you feel you are prepared to leave your current job, you will need to give them adequate notice so they can find your replacement. Otherwise, your clients may not receive the treatment that they expect. In some cases, a company will drop clients if the RBT quits since they did not have anyone to fill in. You certainly do not want to be accused of abandoning your clients.

Code 3.04 Test Yourself: Multiple-Choice Question

1. The agency for which you are working has started to take conduct disorder cases. Your only experience is working with children with autism and providing language training. Your supervisor asked if you have any experience with conduct disorder. How should you respond?
   a. "Sign me up! This is exciting. I have plenty of experience."
   b. "I have more experience with conduct disorder than I do with autism."
   c. "Did you read my résumé? I think my experience would be good."

d. "I would love the opportunity to work with a new population, but I would need training and supervision because I have no experience with conduct disorder."

Code 3.04 Test Yourself: True or False Question

2. The company at which you are working treats young children with ASD, but they are looking to begin working with adolescents diagnosed with oppositional defiant disorder (ODD) and conduct disorder. You've had experience working with one 4-year-old child who had a diagnosis of ASD and feel confident that you can generalize the skills you developed with that client to this teen population without additional assistance. Assuming you can generalize your skills is an ethical approach.
   True or False?
   True
   False

For correct answers, go to Appendix A

3.05 RBTs PROVIDE BEHAVIOR TECHNICIAN SERVICES ONLY WITHIN DEFINED ROLES

Quick Take

"This behavior analysis stuff just doesn't work, I tried it on my husband and he just got mad."

The intent of this Code item is to discourage RBTs from freely giving advice or providing behavior-analytic services to friends, relatives, or neighbors. This can be quite a challenge since once people find out that you have special skills in behavior change, they will want to pick your brain for ideas for their unruly child, their barking dog, or even their spouse who refuses to help with chores around the house. It can be quite flattering to be asked these questions and to be treated like an expert, but to provide answers under these circumstances would be unethical; that is, it could cause long-term harm to someone. There is a very good chance that this very interested but quite untrained person would not be able to follow your advice exactly and will simply make matters worse. Then they likely will blame you for giving bad advice, and finally they may conclude that, "This behavior analysis stuff just doesn't work, I tried it on my husband and he just got mad, yelled at me, and called me manipulative and other names."

CHALLENGE 1: While treating a client in a classroom setting, you frequently consult with the teacher regarding behavior reduction strategies with your client. There are other children in the classroom who also present behavior problems but do not receive any behavioral services. One child frequently engages in yelling out and calling names (you believe this is maintained by attention—the teacher provides attention only when he engages in those behaviors). One day, you noticed the teacher is clearly agitated. She walked over to you and said, "I just don't know what to do with Mason. He just keeps getting worse, and it's disrupting the other students. Do you have any recommendations?"

RBT RESPONSE: "It looks like he's doing this for attention. I know it's really hard, but you have to ignore him when he acts like that."

(One week passes)

TEACHER: "The ignoring didn't work; now he comes over and knocks things off of my desk, then just stands there. He's even worse now than he was before!"

COMMENTARY: This RBT made the wrong call when giving advice to the teacher on a student that was not her client. Although this recommendation may have been given in good faith, she ended up causing more harm than good. *Advice should never be given outside of the defined role of a therapist-provider relationship, regardless of how harmless it may seem*. In a situation like this, it would be better to say, "Unfortunately, I am not able to comment on his behavior, as he is not my client and it would violate my code of ethics. Would you like me to bring in my supervisor?"

CHALLENGE 2: Someone you used to work with sent you a message on Facebook that said, "Hi, I noticed that you do ABA with kids with ASD. My son was recently diagnosed with that. We've been having trouble getting him therapy because the wait lists everywhere here are so long. Do you have any advice on things we can start doing now before he begins therapy?"

WHAT NOT TO SAY: "Sure. Tell me a little more about him, and I can offer some tips on what to do. I've picked up quite a few tips at my new job."

WHAT *TO* SAY: "I'm sorry, I'm afraid I am not able to comment on this. I would have to clear this with my boss first and she is a real stickler for compliance with our ethics code."

COMMENTARY: This is another classic situation RBTs regularly encounter: most people have little experience with effective behavioral treatment and if they find out you have it, they see no reason not to ask for help. In our culture, people like to help others when they ask, and of course they offer often unwanted advice freely as well. A "defined role" is one that includes a signed job contract or written agreement with a company or agency. Offering tips, suggestions, advice, or opinions about behavior treatment to someone

> *"It is a good idea to have a short script ready in case someone catches you at the grocery store or in a bar and starts asking questions and begging for answers."*

on a bus, subway, or plane certainly does not meet the requirement of a *defined role*.

CHALLENGE 3: Along with another RBT, you are providing treatment in a classroom. You each work with different clients. The teacher is particularly difficult and has a history of pressuring RBTs to act unethically.

TEACHER: "I know you've seen how disruptive Juan is when it's time to do worksheets. He's always ripping up the papers and attacking me. What do you think I should do about that?"

RBT 1: "Oh, I'm not really sure. I don't know him all that well."

TEACHER: "Yes, but you do behavior therapy, right? Shouldn't you know how to fix that?"

RBT 1: (looks down, visibly uncomfortable) "Well, you know Juan is not my client."

RBT 2: (gives nod of approval to RBT 1)

RBT 1: "He's not my client and ethically I can't give advice on his behaviors."

TEACHER: "Come on! You have to tell me something."

RBT 2: (Gives another nod of approval)

RBT 1: "No, I'm sorry. That is not something that I can do." (turns attention toward client and away from teacher).

COMMENTARY: Upholding the Code is no small task, but it can be made easier by the support of fellow RBTs. In this case, RBT 2 could have actually spoken up and corroborated RBT 1's position.

More Details

The "defined role" that this code item refers to means a job assignment for which you have a written contract to provide services and where you will be properly supervised by an experienced BCBA. A contract, also known as an agreement, specifies exactly what is expected of you, includes the names of the persons contracted with, gives a beginning and ending date of the assignment, lists the payment you will receive and how often you will be paid, describes what happens if you or the other party breaks the contract, and finally has signature lines and date lines. It is a good idea to have a short script ready in case someone catches you at the grocery store or in a bar and starts asking questions and begging for answers. "I'm sorry; I'm not able to give advice without approval from my agency, and I only work for them," is a good response that you can vary to suit the circumstances. It is true and should help get you out of this awkward situation quickly. Avoid saying anything that could be construed as actual advice ("Have you tried extinction?"), and don't play games by saying, "I'll have to get back with you on that one" or "That's a tough one; let me think on that a while."

Code 3.05 Test Yourself: Multiple-Choice Questions

1. While you were waiting for your client to arrive at school, another student in the classroom started to engage in a tantrum. He was throwing desks and chairs and was becoming aggressive toward peers in the classroom. The teacher began begging you to "Do your RBT behavior thing!" with this child. How should you have responded?
   a. "Yes, I can definitely help, but once my client is here, I will have to go to him."
   b. "I'm sorry but I'm not allowed to intervene with this child, but I can call the office and get some help."
   c. "I'm sorry; I only work with one student at a time."
   d. "Oh, sorry; I think I see my client walking in."
2. A long-time friend got a new puppy and was struggling to house-train Daisy and teach her basic commands. Your friend came to you for advice, saying, "You're the RBT and do behavior change stuff all day. Can't you help me?" How should you respond?
   a. "You're the one that got a puppy; you should have thought about that before getting one."

b. "My job is working with humans, not animals. Changing animal behavior would be different."
c. "I'm sorry, but would be unethical for me to give that kind of advice. I've never even owned a dog."
d. "There's a little thing called reinforcement; you could look into that."

3. One day a parent asked you for advice on a behavior problem she was having with her daughter Lily. You treat her son, Theo, but are not contracted to provide services to Lily. How should you respond?
   a. "You remember the ABC data sheets we used before with Theo? Just fill out one of those when it occurs so I can get a better idea of what's going on."
   b. "Hmmm, let me think about this. I will get back to you."
   c. "Have you tried running the same protocol that we used with Theo? This sounds pretty similar, and you could do this on your own."
   d. "Unfortunately, I am not allowed to advise on Lily's behaviors as she technically isn't our client."

Code 3.05 Test Yourself: True or False Questions

4. As you were leaving a home session, your client's mom stopped you and asked about prompting mands. She wanted to make sure she was doing the same thing as you and wanted to know how to motivate her child. You explained to mom the procedures you are using and told her to contact the BCBA if she would like some parent training or if she has questions about the mand program. This was a good way of handling this situation.
   True or False?
   True
   False
5. You have a cousin with autism, and you will periodically give your aunt and uncle tips on things such as using

reinforcement, responding to tantrums, and improving his communication skills. You would never go as far as to write an actual protocol or offer any extensive treatment recommendations, but sometimes your relatives call when they are having issues and you give them advice. Giving these tips is okay since they are relatives.

True or False?

True

False

For correct answers, go to Appendix A

3.06 WHEN RBTs PROVIDE SERVICES, THEY COMMUNICATE WITH CLIENTS IN A SIMPLE AND EASY-TO-UNDERSTAND WAY

Quick Take

> *"When communicating with clients, however, we have to be careful to speak a language that they use and understand."*

Our behavior analysis technology is full of jargon that we love to use when talking to each other: *reinforcement, extinction, DRO, fading, contingency, time-out*, and many other technical terms define our field. Technical talk allows us to make important distinctions that can make a difference in whether a procedure changes a behavior effectively or actually makes things worse. When communicating with clients, however, we have to be careful to speak a language that they use and understand.

Compare this: "Ms. Jones, it is really important that you maintain consistency in the delivery of the reinforcer in order to strengthen Brian's operant compliance behavior" with "Ms. Jones, remember to give Brian his reward every time he does what you asked him to do."

Here are some common terms and English translations:

Aversive	Disliked stimulus or activity
Chaining	One behavior leads to another
Contingency	If-then statements, consequences for behavior
DRO	Reward some *other* behavior
Escape-maintained	Get out of something they don't like
Extinction	Planned ignoring of a specific behavior
Motivating Operation	A change that makes something rewarding
Response Effort	Make something hard to do
Reinforcement	Reward for a specific behavior
Timeout	Move to a quiet place where no reward is available

CHALLENGE 1: When he engages in his schoolwork, your client receives tokens that you deliver. His teacher asks how the system works; she wants to implement it during the times when a therapist is not there. You explain, "Provide a token contingent on task completion on a variable-interval schedule of 3 minutes, but implement the response cost when he engages in problem behavior." The next time you come for the client's session, you see that he has no tokens and is having a full-blown emotional outburst. The teacher says that he was talking without raising his hand, so he lost all of his tokens and that the token board doesn't work for him.

RBT RESPONSE: "Oh no, that's not what I meant. It's not working because he loses his tokens for off-task behavior, not because he didn't raise his hand; plus, he should only lose one at a time, but has to earn it back quickly."

TEACHER RESPONSE: "That is NOT what you said. I was trying to give him the tokens every three minutes like you said, but he was not completing his work fast enough and I needed to move on. Then he started crying and talking without raising his hand, so I took the tokens. I will be contacting your supervisor about this."

COMMENTARY: Getting teacher buy-in is one of the hardest tasks of working in a classroom. This RBT should have translated the vocabulary into plain English and then met with the BCBA about some teacher training.

CHALLENGE 2: At drop-off, you are talking with a mom who says, "How is my son doing with his picture naming?"

RBT RESPONSE: "His what? Oh, do you mean his tacting program?"

MOTHER RESPONSE: "Um, I'm not sure. Is that the one where you show him pictures and he says what it is?"

RBT RESPONSE: "Oh yes that's it. It's called tacting and we're using it to help build some of his expressive language skills. He's doing great by the way; he's at 100% accuracy on all his targets with a partial vocal, verbal prompt!"

MOTHER RESPONSE: "A partial what?"

COMMENTARY This RBT took the jargon of ABA too far in her conversation with a parent. It is important to gauge the parent's knowledge and use language that matches their understanding. Using this type of language is also problematic as it may distance the parent from therapy and disenchant them.

> *"Remember, your goal is not to teach the caregivers our language but instead to use their common vocabulary to teach them to understand the fundamentals of behavior."*

More Details

Most of our technical vocabulary came out of the early animal labs that Skinner set up when he was a graduate student at Harvard University in 1931–1936 and then later when he returned as a professor from 1948 to 1974. Skinner studied the operant behavior of rats and pigeons and developed the terminology to communicate with his students and colleagues, and we have kept most of that vocabulary to this day. While he was very interested in the applications of this science of behavior to the human condition, he did not live to see the proliferation of amazing, effective therapies that we take for granted today. As an RBT, you need to learn this terminology to understand applied behavior analysis in all of its complexity and to be able to communicate with your supervisor and other BCBAs that you will encounter. However, it is not a good idea to try to impress the family of your clients or a classroom teacher with your proficiency by tossing around terms like continuous reinforcement, conditioned reinforcers, fixed-ratio schedule, or extinction. Rather, they are more likely to be put off by what they may consider mere jargon with little purpose. Our advice is to practice making translations of operant language into plain English in every conversation. Remember, your goal is not to teach the caregivers *our* language but instead to use their common vocabulary to teach them to understand the fundamentals of behavior.

Code 3.06 Test Yourself: Multiple-Choice Questions

1. You are working on completing homework tasks with your client. At the end of the session, her mother stops you and asks for instructions on how to get Camila to complete her homework when you aren't there. How should you respond?
   a. "It's simple and it works like this . . . contingent on work completion and accuracy of 80% or higher, Camila earns a reinforcer of her choice. This is typically watching

a video on her tablet, but she is only allowed two minutes prior to beginning the next page of homework. However, contingent on problem behavior, she does not earn the reinforcer."

b. "When Camila finishes her homework and it is fairly accurate, she can earn a few minutes on her tablet watching videos. If she cries, screams, or leaves the table, she doesn't earn the tablet and we move on to the next assignment."

c. "Contingencies like this are hard to explain."

d. "It is somewhat technical and involves manipulating the environment ahead of time."

2. One of the teachers in a classroom where you are working with a client has started letting your client take a "calm down" break every time he engages in problem behaviors during work time. This involves allowing him to escape the task and access preferred items, plus attention from the teacher's aide. Which of the following is the best way to discuss this with the teacher?

   a. "You need to put those behaviors on extinction, or this is just going to get worse."

   b. "So, we have this principle called primary functions of behaviors. They include escape from demands, access to tangibles, and social attention. It looks like you are doing a few of them right now, but you could be making his problem behaviors worse."

   c. "How about you just use Functional Communication Training (FCT) to allow him escape from demands and access to tangibles?"

   d. "Can you explain how these 'calm down' breaks work? A concern I have is that by giving him a break from work and giving him toys after he engages in inappropriate behavior, we might be making his behaviors worse. Let me talk to my supervisor and see if we can help create a program to work on it."

Code 3.06 Test Yourself: True or False Question

3. It is the responsibility of the RBT to educate teachers and caregivers on the proper ABA terminology to ensure that there is consistency and accuracy in communicating behavior analytic treatment. This tactic is appropriate and ethical.
   True or False?
   True
   False

For correct answers, go to Appendix A

3.07 RBTs COLLECT AND DISPLAY DATA IN A WAY THAT ALLOWS FOR DECISIONS AND RECOMMENDATIONS TO BE MADE FOR PROGRAM DEVELOPMENT

> *"Accurate data collection and clear graphic representation are so important that carrying out these tasks inappropriately is considered unethical by the Certification Board."*

Quick Take

The central, pivotal role of the RBT in the data collection process cannot be overestimated. If the data you collect is not accurate or reliable, then decisions made by your ABA team will be faulty, and your client could suffer the consequences. The team reviewing the data will be making decisions about whether to continue or phase out a treatment or possibly increase or decrease a medication dosage (in conjunction with the client's physician). A lot is at stake with data collection, since as an evidence-based field, we depend on the data collected by RBTs, and we assume that it is rock solid and dependable over a long period of treatment. Insurance companies and Medicaid rely heavily on behavioral-based data to determine whether funding will be continued or dropped or possibly increased depending on the trends over time.

Likewise, graphing of that data must be accurately displayed and easily interpreted so that day-to-day decisions can be made regarding trending or phase changes, such as when a determination is made, for example, that a behavior has reached a plateau. Accurate data collection and clear graphic representation are so important that carrying out these tasks inappropriately is considered *unethical* by the Certification Board.

CHALLENGE 1: For months, you have been working on a tooth-brushing program with your client. He has made a lot of progress and most of the time can brush his teeth independently, but he still has days where he requires additional prompting. When he does make errors, it seems to be because he just doesn't want to do it, not because he can't do it. You feel like there are more important things on which you could be working. Honestly, you're just tired of running this program. Unfortunately, the mastery criteria is 100% independence for five consecutive sessions, and although he often gets close to this, his graph shows that he is falling short of this goal.

RBT RESPONSE: Prior to the session, you looked at the client's graph for the past few days and determined that he was right around 85% independence. When you ran the program, the client needed a little prompting, but you decided to just graph the data at 100%.

COMMENTARY: Deliberate falsification of data is certainly unethical and can create a lot of problems for you *and* your client. Your supervisor, the parents, and others make important decisions based on graphs of client data. When having concerns regarding a program, you should always bring it to the attention of your supervisor rather than faking data and graphing it.

CHALLENGE 2: As Randy's primary therapist, over the last two years, you have watched him make tremendous progress. You met with your supervisor to discuss Randy's case, and the supervisor said, "Isn't it amazing how far

Randy has come? Remember when he first started and all he could say was 'No'? Now he's mastered most of the VB-MAPP. As soon as we finish up these last few objectives, he'll be ready for fade out and discharge."

RBT: Although you know you should be happy for Randy, the thought of no longer seeing him is depressing, so you mark a few trials as incorrect (when they really were correct) so he scores just below mastery criteria, and you prepare the graphs accordingly. You start looking for other skills to pitch to your supervisor that you think your client needs.

COMMENTARY: Saying goodbye to a client you've worked with for a long time can be an incredibly difficult part of this job. Although hard, fading and then discharge is a critical moment for our clients that should be celebrated and encouraged by the team members. Sabotaging the process through miscalculation of data and showing non-representative graphs only hinders the independence of the client and delays much-needed services to children on the waitlist. Even more serious, deliberate falsification of data is not only unethical but also illegal since it is connected to billing and could be considered fraud.

> *"Graphs should be easy for your supervisor to understand and interpret so that decisions can be made and recommendations put forward for behavior programming."*

More Details

As an RBT, you may be required to collect data using continuous or discontinuous measurement procedures or record permanent product outcomes. The decision on which system to use will usually be made by your BCBA supervisor. You may have been provided with training by your agency, clinic, or company in the data collection conventions they have adopted, so you will be expected to follow those guidelines. Some companies have gone with electronic computer-based data collection systems such as Catalyst or Central Reach, in which case you will be using an iPad or tablet provided by your company. This device will be pre-programmed with the target behaviors and will be set up with measurement systems such as frequency, duration, partial- or whole-interval or momentary time sampling already built in. The bottom line for data collection is that it must be accurate and reliable. Reliability is determined by Inter-Observer Agreement (IOA) checks you should do with your supervisor on a regular basis.

When it comes to graphing, all of the same considerations apply. Your supervisor will probably show you how she likes to see graphs prepared so they are easy to understand, and your company may have standard conventions that they have adopted. If they are using dedicated iPads or tablets, these may also have graphing built in, and you will probably require training in how to generate graphs. Graphs should be easy for your supervisor to understand and interpret so that decisions can be made and recommendations put forward for behavior programming. Standard graphing conventions used by the *Journal of Applied Behavior Analysis* can be seen subsequently.

Code 3.07 Test Yourself: Multiple-Choice Question

1. Your company uses an electronic data collection system where data is entered on a tablet. When you bring your client outside to the playground, you often leave your tablet inside because it is difficult to carry while running around. At times, the tablet will overheat in the sun, which makes it shut down for extended periods. How can you maintain appropriate data collection?
   a. The tablet must be with you at all times. Providing therapy without it would be a violation.

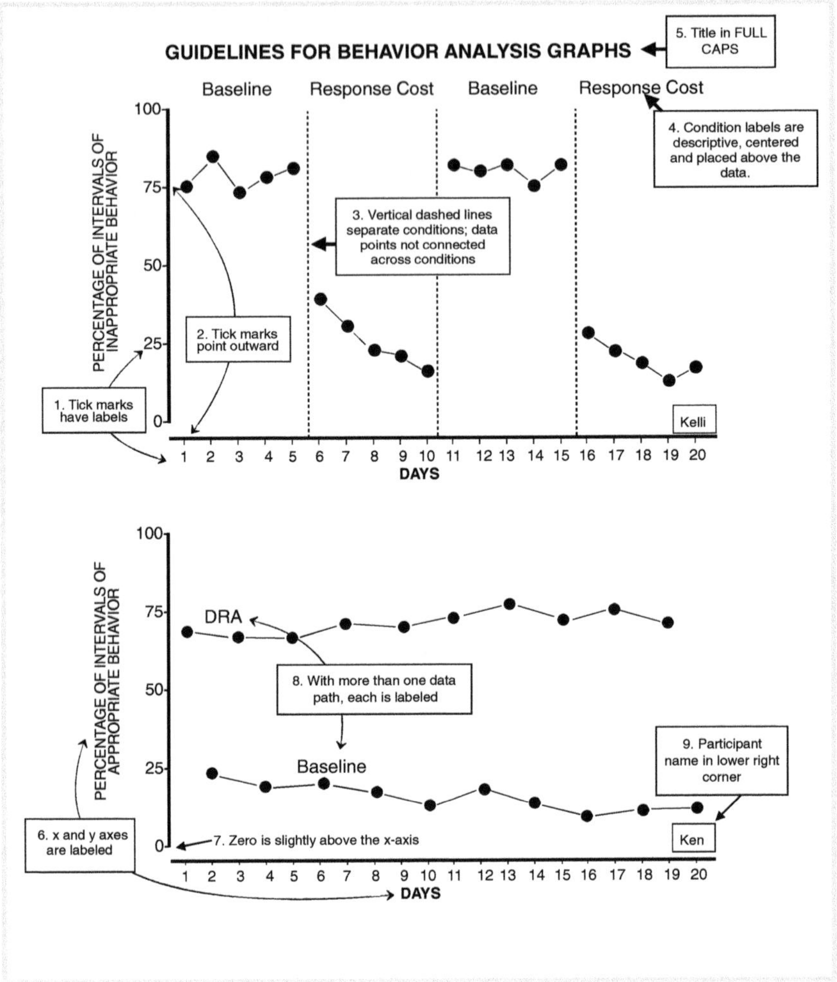

Figure 6.1 Guidelines for Behavior Analysis Graphs
Source: Reused with permission from Taylor & Francis

b. Record an estimate of data when returning inside.
c. Do not record any behavior that occurred during that time.
d. Discuss with your supervisor other ways of collecting that would be appropriate to use during that time.

Test Yourself: True or False Questions

2. The client you are working with engages in severe aggression. The data collection specifies that aggression will be collected in 30 s episodes. After 30 s, should the client aggress again, then that aggression would get recorded, but not if it occurred within the 30 s. You know this client engages in frequent aggression, but this data collection makes the aggression appear it is not as frequent as it is. You start recording *every instance* of aggression despite the training you received. This is acceptable and follows Code 3.07.
   True or False?
   True
   False
3. Your clinic is using a new graphing program, and the BCBAs are still learning how to use it. You have experience working with this program, so you decide to create a mock graph showing how the graphs would look and offer to help make the new graphs. This is not a violation of 3.07.
   True or False?
   True
   False
4. The behavior program for one of your clients requires that you track many behaviors. You find it difficult to memorize all the behavior definitions and sometimes forget specific details like whether tears need to be present to mark crying or the inter-response time between tantrums to designate a new episode. While conducting treatment, you just use your judgment on tracking behavior. It is unethical to just use your own judgment in this situation.
   True or False?
   True
   False

For correct answers, go to Appendix A

3.08 IF RBTs ARE INVOLVED IN THE DELIVERY OF NON-BEHAVIOR-ANALYTIC INTERVENTIONS, THEY DO NOT MAKE REFERENCE TO, DISPLAY, OR OTHERWISE USE THEIR RBT IN THAT PRACTICE

> *"Behavior analysts do not implement non-behavior-analytic interventions."*

Quick Take

The purpose of this code item is to prevent *any association* of our well-researched behavior-analytic treatments with the vast number of non-behavior-analytic methods that are currently popular in our culture. We don't want the public to think these other non-evidence-based treatments are approved by or used by behavior analysts, since this would ultimately debase our reputation as behavioral scientists.

The Professional and Ethical Compliance Code for Behavior Analysts (a.k.a. the BCBA Code, or the Code) has a strong statement on this issue, Code 8.01 (b), which says, "Behavior analysts do *not* implement non-behavior-analytic interventions" (italics added), and we believe that this position is the proper standard for our field.

So, how might an RBT become "involved in the delivery of non-behavior-analytic interventions"? This could happen, for example, if you were working with a family that, prior to signing up for ABA treatment, was involved in taking their child to the Florida Keys twice a year for dolphin-assisted therapy. They invite you to go along and offer to pay for your room and board if you will help their son Lucas get in and out of the pool and not have tantrums if the dolphin comes up to him. After telling the family that this is *not* a behavior-analytic treatment and discussing the matter with your supervisor, if you end up in Key Largo, you would not present yourself as an RBT to the dolphin therapist but rather just say, "I'm Lucas's friend, and I'm here to help."

It is important to add that it would be inappropriate to bill for any non-behavior-analytic treatment even if it *was* implemented by an RBT.

CHALLENGE 1: You have been treating Avery, a 6-year-old, for food selectivity by using a shaping procedure. Currently the program entails placing a piece of carrot on the plate and using a DRO for the absence of inappropriate behaviors.

RBT RESPONSE: You see how upset Avery can get and have been thinking about other things you can do to make the procedure less aversive. During your next session, you bring your essential oils with you and put a drop on her forehead to help relieve stress before you bring out the carrot. When she starts to get upset, you hold her hand and take her over to the corner of the room and have her practice a calming yoga pose that always makes you feel better when you are agitated or upset.

COMMENTARY: Your role as a behavior analyst is strictly to perform behavior analytic services. Although this RBT had good intentions, using non-behavior analytic interventions while practicing as an RBT is strictly prohibited.

CHALLENGE 2: Trevor, a school client, receives occupational therapy from the district therapist. Trevor sees the OT twice a week for 15 minutes. He sometimes engages in severe aggression, including toward the OT. The OT has asked you to start putting a weighted blanket on Trevor every time he aggresses. The OT tells you that Trevor clearly needs some sensory input and is getting this from aggressing. She believes if you put the blanket on him, he won't lash out toward adults anymore.

WHAT NOT TO DO: You aren't sure how you are supposed to respond, so you tell the OT that you will try your best to use the blanket, but that's not really what your protocol is.

WHAT *TO* DO: You know you are only allowed to implement behavior-analytic procedures, so you tell the OT that you will need to talk to your supervisor before making any changes to the protocol.

COMMENTARY: It can be extremely uncomfortable to deny a recommendation from another professional, especially someone who is more credentialed than you. However, as an RBT in the field of ABA, you are ethically bound to implement only behavior-analytic interventions. There is not a lot of applied behavioral research supporting the use of a weighted blanket, and it's possible that this would reinforce the client's problem behavior. It's best to have a "go to" response for these situations, such as, "Here is my BCBA's number if you want to run this by her."

CHALLENGE 3: A parent told you when she was picking up her child at your clinic that she purchased a hyperbaric oxygen therapy chamber for home use, but her son Benjie really doesn't like it. She said most of the time, she cannot even get him into the chamber and asked if you could assist her since you work so well with Benjie at the clinic.

RBT RESPONSE: "Unfortunately, because that isn't a behavior-analytic treatment, it's not something I can do."

PARENT RESPONSE: "Oh, you wouldn't have to do any of the therapy, the machine does all of that; all you need to do is help get him into it."

RBT RESPONSE: "Let me ask my supervisor and see what he says."

> *"The standard test for a behavior-analytic treatment is to ask if research on the method has been published in JABA."*

COMMENTARY: Parents of children with behavioral problems are sometimes desperate and willing to try just about anything. An RBT certainly cannot assist with this therapy, but you should also pass this along to the supervisor so that she can help educate the parents on the use of evidence-based treatments.

More Details

To qualify as a behavior-analytic treatment, the intervention has to meet the requirements specified by Baer, Wolf, and Risley (1968) in their classic paper, "The Current Dimensions of Applied Behavior Analysis," which include applied, behavioral, analytic, technological, conceptual, effective, and generalization. The standard test for a behavior-analytic treatment is to ask if research on the method has been published in the *Journal of Applied Behavior Analysis* (*JABA*).

The list of non-evidence-based treatments for ASD is very long and includes such treatments as facilitated communication, prism glasses, holding therapy, chelation, hyperbaric oxygen therapy, gluten free-casein free diet, vitamin supplements, raw camel milk, transcranial magnetic stimulation, DIR Floortime, Zones of Regulation, and, practically beyond belief, bleach therapy. In addition, there are serious questions about the therapeutic effects of some occupational therapy treatments such as weighted vests and brushing. An excellent reference for further details can be found in a recent chapter by Dr. Bruce Thyer entitled "Pseudoscientific Therapies for Autism Spectrum Disorder" (see references subsequently).

Code 3.08 Test Yourself: Multiple-Choice Questions

1. When you were reviewing a client's programs, you noticed there was a new one called "Identifying Zones." You read through the program and saw the purpose is for emotional and sensory self-management. While "The Zones" is used in his classroom, you have never implemented this with your client. The teacher prompts the client to identify the

zones. You feel certain this is not a behavior-analytic protocol. How you should respond/act?

a. Don't say anything, but do not run the program when you are with the client.
b. Find a time to talk to your BCBA about the program and see if she can explain why you are teaching something that is not an ABA treatment.
c. Leave the programs on your BCBA's desk with a note saying you won't work with this client until that unethical program is taken out.
d. Write a strongly worded email to your BCBA, clinical director, and agency owner about how unethical the agency is.

2. A parent asks you to begin using a brushing technique with your client because the OT has been using it, and the mother feels it has been effective at reducing his aggression. How should you respond?
   a. "I've heard that's a hoax. I can't believe you are using this."
   b. "Okay, we can give it a try and see how it goes."
   c. "We're only allowed to use behavior-analytic interventions, so I don't think we will be able use it. Let me check with my supervisor and see what she says."
   d. "I'm sure we can make that work. I just might have to change a few things to make it more behavior analytic."

Code 3.08 Test Yourself: True or False Question

3. One of your clients is severely allergic to gluten (he has a doctor's note), so he is on a gluten-free diet. His parents want to work on teaching the client to identify things he can and can't eat. You and your BCBA work together on

creating an "allergy identifying" program. This does not conflict with the Code.

True or False?

True

False

For correct answers, go to Appendix A

FOR FURTHER READING

https://autismsciencefoundation.org/what-is-autism/beware-of-non-evidence-based-treatments/

Thyer, B. A. (2019). Pseudoscientific therapies for Autism spectrum disorder. In J. L. Matson (Ed.), *Handbook of Intellectual Disabilities, Autism and Child Psychopathology*. New York: Springer Nature Switzerland.

7

RBT Responsibilities to the Board

This section is comparable to section 10 in the BACB Professional and Ethical Compliance Code for Behavior Analysts, where the Code lays out the rules for informing the Board about their applications and any changes to their status. 1) RBTs are advised to be truthful in providing this information, 2) to inform the Board if there are any changes to their status, such as legal charges, disciplinary actions, or physical or mental impairments that might affect their work, and are also advised to inform the Board of any changes in their name or address. 3) Since RBTs might be required to prepare materials for clients or their agencies, they are warned against using the BACB's IP, which includes all of their copyrights and trademarked materials and logo. 4) RBTs will be involved in testing, and they are reminded of their obligation to be honest in providing information and warned against cheating in any manner. 5) Finally, RBTs are prompted to comply with all BACB requirements for training, assessments, audits, and supervision.

In addition to the specific code elements given previously, all RBTs and RBT applicants must:

1. Provide truthful and accurate information to the BACB. *This includes any applications or documentation submitted to the BACB.*

2. Report the following to the BACB within 30 days: legal charges (and subsequent related actions and documents as requested by the BACB); investigations and disciplinary actions by employers (e.g., suspensions and terminations for cause), governmental agencies, educational institutions, and third-party payers; a physical or mental condition that impairs the RBT's ability to safely work; or a change of name, mailing address, or email address. *If you have any doubt about whether you should report some information, check the BACB.com site for details; when in doubt, report anyway just to be safe.*
3. Adhere to all requirements regarding use of BACB intellectual property (see 10.03 of the *Professional and Ethical Compliance Code for Behavior Analysts*). *This is a very extensive list, so review it closely if you have any question as to whether you might be infringing on BACB intellectual property.*
4. Adhere to the rules of the BACB and approved testing centers, including, but not limited to, rules related to cheating; falsifying information; and unauthorized collection, use, or distribution of exam materials. *Refer to 10.04 of the BACB Code for details on examination honesty and irregularities.*
5. Comply with all BACB requirements for RBT training, assessment, audits, and supervision. *See BACB Code 10.05 for details and also Code 5.0 with regard to supervision.*

CHALLENGE 1: An applicant for the RBT makes an appointment to take the examination at a Pearson Professional Center. As she steps out of her Honda, she is approached by a well-dressed young man, who whispers, "I can guarantee you will pass the exam. I've got the answers right here (he shows her a small folded-up piece of paper). It's a bargain at $25; I only take cash, though."

PRE-RBT RESPONSE: "I'm sorry; I'm not interested—get out of here (she whips her phone out of her back pocket, turns and snaps a photo of the guy and his car, and memorizes his license plate as he pulls away)."

COMMENTARY: This applicant will make an excellent RBT. She knew that it would be dishonest to buy the answers and acted quickly to try to get some information that might lead to his capture.

CHALLENGE 2: In his first week of work as an RBT, Ryan had a run-in with a local sheriff's deputy. He was pulled over for a broken tail light, but a misunderstanding ensued about what exactly the deputy wanted. The next thing Ryan knew, he got a ticket for refusing to disclose his name. Ryan was shaken; he had a perfect driving record and didn't know what to do. An attorney friend said he could get him out of the ticket, but he would have to appear before a judge in two weeks to explain what happened. In all the confusion, Ryan completely forgot to inform the Board about the incident.

COMMENTARY: This could be a serious violation, and at this point, Ryan's only option is to immediately inform the Board of what happened and beg forgiveness, understanding that there may be some sort of penalty.

CHALLENGE 3: Ainslee moved for the third time in six months. This time, she signed a 1-year lease, so this move felt permanent. Ainslee just signed on with a new multiservice agency as a brand new RBT and was excited to get started working with kids again. Her new supervisor asked her about her new apartment, and Ainslee mentioned that she could see the Space Needle from her kitchen window.

SUPERVISOR RESPONSE: "Speaking of a new address, by the way, did you inform the Board about your new address?"

RBT RESPONSE: "Oh, no, I completely forgot. Is it too late? What do I need to do?"

SUPERVISOR: "Well, you know you are supposed to report any change of address within 30 days."

COMMENTARY: It's understandable that Ainslee would forget about letting the Board know of her new address, but she is nonetheless responsible for keeping the Board updated in case they need to get in touch with her.

Part

Three

Answers to Test-Yourself Questions, the RBT Ethics Code, Glossary, and Scripts and Conversation Starters

Appendix A: Answers to Test-Yourself Questions

Code 1.01

1. B
2. C
3. A
4. False

Code 1.02

1. A
2. C
3. B
4. False

Code 1.03

1. B
2. B

3. D
4. C
5. True

Code 1.04

1. D
2. B
3. C

Code 1.05

1. C
2. A
3. B

Code 1.06

1. B
2. A
3. True
4. False

Code 1.07

1. C
2. True
3. False

Code 1.08

1. C
2. False

Code 1.09

1. B
2. C
3. D
4. Yes

Code 1.10

1. B
2. False

Code 1.11

1. B
2. C
3. False; this violates Code 1.11: you misrepresented the intensity of the workshop.

Code 1.12

1. A
2. True
3. False

Code 1.13

1. C
2. D
3. C
4. True

Code 2.01

1. C
2. False
3. True
4. False

Code 2.02

1. D
2. C
3. A
4. False
5. True

Code 2.03

1. C
2. True
3. True

Code 2.04

1. D
2. C
3. True
4. False
5. False

Code 2.05

1. A
2. D
3. True
4. True

Code 2.06

1. C
2. B
3. False

Code 2.07

1. D
2. A
3. **False**. You will want to follow up with your supervisor about the bruises you observed. It is likely that you will have to file a report with your agency and your state's child protective services. As an RBT, you are a mandated reporter. That means that if you see something (bruises, poor hygiene, little food, etc.) that indicates that your

client might not be in a safe environment, then you are ethically and legally bound to report what you saw.
4. True

Code 2.08

1. A
2. B
3. D
4. False
5. True

Code 2.09

1. B
2. B
3. False
4. False
5. True

Code 2.10

1. **False**. It might be beneficial to utilize a cover sheet for data sheets or a clamshell clipboard so confidential information is not available for all to see.

Code 3.01

1. B
2. D
3. False
4. True

Code 3.02

1. C
2. A

3. True
4. False
5. True

Code 3.03

1. C
2. True
3. False
4. True

Code 3.04

1. D
2. False

Code 3.05

1. B
2. C
3. D
4. True
5. False

Code 3.06

1. B
2. D
3. False

Code 3.07

1. D. In behavior analysis, we rely heavily on accurate data collection to make treatment decisions. At times, our data collection methods may interfere with our ability to record accurate data. If your supervisor does not frequently conduct therapy, she may not be aware of some of these issues, so it is always best to discuss any concerns you have. In

a situation like this, maybe it makes more sense to use a clicker or pen-and-paper recording.

2. False
3. True
4. True

Code 3.08

1. B
2. C
3. True

Appendix B: The RBT Ethics Code

The RBT Ethics Code describes the ethical requirements for both RBTs and RBT applicants. All RBTs and RBT applicants must agree to abide by this code. Because RBTs are not independent practitioners and must receive ongoing supervision of their practice, those who supervise RBTs must also be familiar with this code.

In addition to the specific code elements subsequently, all RBTs and RBT applicants must:

- provide truthful and accurate information to the BACB;
- report the following to the BACB within 30 days: legal charges (and subsequent related actions and documents as requested by the BACB); investigations and disciplinary actions by employers (e.g., suspensions and terminations for cause), governmental agencies, educational institutions, and third-party payers; a physical or mental condition that impairs the RBT's ability to safely work; or a change of name, mailing address, or email address;

- adhere to all requirements regarding use of BACB intellectual property (see 10.03 of the *Professional and Ethical Compliance Code for Behavior Analysts*);
- adhere to the rules of the BACB and approved testing centers, including, but not limited to, rules related to cheating; falsifying information; and unauthorized collection, use, or distribution of exam materials; and
- comply with all BACB requirements for RBT training, assessment, audits, and supervision.

SECTION 1—RESPONSIBLE CONDUCT

The RBT Ethics Code includes 31 items that encompass basic values and core principles that should be adhered to by technicians and therapists operating in clinics, schools, and in-home settings.

1.01 RBTs uphold and promote the values and core principles of behavior analysis.

1.02 RBTs have an obligation to remain familiar with this code. Lack of knowledge or understanding of this code does not excuse unethical conduct.

1.03 RBTs are truthful and honest and create an environment that promotes truthful and honest behavior in others. They promote an ethical culture in their work environments and make others aware of this code.

1.04 RBTs act in a way that conforms to the legal and ethical codes of the professional and social communities where they are members. They do not lead others to engage in fraudulent, illegal, or unethical conduct.

1.05 If RBTs' ethical responsibilities conflict with employer policies, RBTs must bring the conflict to their supervisor's attention, document that they did so, and document the resolution.

1.06 RBTs avoid multiple relationships with clients and supervisors. If they find that a multiple relationship has developed due to unforeseen circumstances, they inform their supervisor and work to resolve it. If the multiple relationship involves their supervisor, the RBT should report it to the person to whom their supervisor reports.

1.07 RBTs do not engage in sexual relationships with clients or supervisors. RBTs refrain from sexual relationships with former clients or supervisors for at least two (2) years following the date the working relationship ended.

1.08 RBTs recognize that their personal problems and conflicts with others may impact their ability to perform their duties and refrain from providing services when this is the case.

1.09 RBTs follow through on obligations and contractual commitments with high quality work and they do not make commitments they cannot keep.

1.10 RBTs do not make false, deceptive, misleading, exaggerated, or fraudulent public statements about their work or qualifications.

1.11 RBTs provide a current and accurate set of credentials (e.g., degrees, certifications) to clients, employers, and supervisors upon request. Changes to certification status must be immediately reported to employers and supervisors.

1.12 RBTs obtain permission to use trademarked or copyrighted materials as required by law. RBTs provide citations that recognize the intellectual property of others, including trademark and copyright symbols.

1.13 RBTs attempt to resolve issues informally when possible, without violating confidentiality, by first bringing the issue to the attention of their supervisor and then the individual involved. RBTs document their efforts to address any of these issues. If the matter cannot be resolved informally, they report it to the appropriate authority (e.g., employer, director, regulatory authority). If the matter meets the reporting requirements of the BACB, RBTs must submit a formal complaint to the BACB.

SECTION 2—RESPONSIBILITY TO CLIENTS

2.01 RBTs support the legal rights and preferences of clients.

2.02 If RBTs become aware that a client's legal rights are being violated, or if there is risk of harm, RBTs must take the necessary action to protect the client. This includes but is not limited to: (1) contacting relevant authorities; (2) following organizational policies; (3) consulting with their supervisor; and (4) documenting their efforts to address the matter.

2.03 When providing services, RBTs do not discriminate against, demean, or harass individuals or groups on the basis of age, gender, race, culture, ethnicity, national origin, religion, sexual orientation, disability, language, socioeconomic status, or any other basis forbidden by law. RBTs recognize their own limitations and obtain the proper training, consultation, or supervision when providing behavior technician services to protected individuals or groups.

2.04 RBTs do not accept gifts from or give gifts to clients.

2.05 RBTs may not share identifying information about clients on social media. They must avoid creating situations where such information could be shared by others, including, but not limited to, written information, photos, or videos.

2.06 RBTs always obtain permission from clients and staff to record interviews and service delivery sessions. Consent must be specifically and separately obtained from each individual.

2.07 RBTs protect the confidentiality and privacy of their clients. RBTs only use relevant identifying information in their job-related communications (e.g., consultation, emails, reports). Confidentiality and privacy requirements may be established by law or by an organization's policies.

2.08 RBTs only discuss confidential information with those who need to know that information. They share information for job-related purposes only. Confidential information includes, but is not limited to: (1) information about anyone with whom the RBT works; or (2) information about anyone to whom the RBT provides services. RBTs maintain confidentiality when handling records under their control. This includes records that are written, electronic, or in any other format. Handling a record may include creation, storage, access, transfer, or disposal.

2.09 RBTs never disclose confidential information without consent from the client. Exceptions are made as required by law, or where allowed by law for a valid reason. This includes, but is not limited to: (1) providing needed services; (2) obtaining appropriate consultations; and (3) protecting the client or others from harm.

2.10 RBTs create, maintain, distribute, store, retain, and dispose of records and data relating to their services (1) in accordance with applicable laws, regulations, and policies; (2) in a way that complies with the requirements of this code; and (3) in a manner that allows for appropriate transition of service at any given time.

SECTION 3—COMPETENCE AND SERVICE DELIVERY

3.01 RBTs only practice under the close, ongoing supervision of a qualified supervisor.

3.02 RBTs follow the direction of their supervisors and inform them when they are asked to do something that goes beyond the scope of their certification.

3.03 RBTs must be competent in the areas in which they provide behavior technician services.

3.04 RBTs may not practice with new client populations without proper training and oversight.

3.05 RBTs provide behavior technician services only within defined roles.

3.06 When RBTs provide services, they communicate with clients in a simple and easy-to-understand way.

3.07 RBTs collect and display data in a way that allows for decisions and recommendations to be made for program development.

3.08 If RBTs are involved in the delivery of non-behavior-analytic interventions, they do not make reference to, display, or otherwise use their RBT in that practice.

Approved by the BACB's Board of Directors on December 17, 2018. This document should be referenced as follows: Behavior Analyst Certification Board®. (2018). RBT® ethics code. Littleton, CO: Author.

Appendix C: Glossary of Behavioral Terms

Provided by the BACB

BEHAVIOR ANALYST

Behavior analyst refers to an individual who holds the BCBA or BCaBA credential, an individual authorized by the BACB to provide supervision, or a coordinator of BACB Approved Course Sequences. Where Code elements are deemed relevant to the practice of an RBT, the term "behavior analyst" includes the behavior technician.

BEHAVIOR-ANALYTIC SERVICES

Behavior-analytic services are those that are explicitly based on principles and procedures of behavior analysis (i.e., the science of behavior) and are designed to change behavior in socially important ways. These services include, but are not limited to, treatment, assessment, training, consultation, managing and supervising others, teaching, and delivering continuing education.

BEHAVIOR-CHANGE PROGRAM

The behavior-change program is a formal, written document that describes in technological detail every assessment and treatment task necessary to achieve stated goals.

CLIENT

The term client refers to any recipient or beneficiary of the professional services provided by a behavior analyst. The term includes, but is not limited to:

1. The direct recipient of services;
2. The parent, relative, legal representative, or legal guardian of the recipient of services;
3. The employer, agency representative, institutional representative, or third-party contractor for services of the behavior analyst; and/or
4. Any other individual or entity that is a known beneficiary of services or who would normally be construed as a "client" or "client-surrogate" in a health-care context.

For purposes of this definition, the term client does not include third-party insurers or payers, unless the behavior analyst is hired directly under contract with the third-party insurer or payer.

FUNCTIONAL ASSESSMENT

Functional assessment, also known as functional behavior assessment, refers to a category of procedures used to formally assess the possible environmental causes of problem behavior. These procedures include informant assessments (e.g., interviews, rating scales), direct observation in the natural environment (e.g., ABC assessment), and experimental functional analysis.

MULTIPLE RELATIONSHIPS

A multiple relationship is one in which a behavior analyst is in both a behavior-analytic role and a non-behavior-analytic role simultaneously with a client or someone closely associated with or related to the client.

PUBLIC STATEMENTS

Public statements include, but are not limited to, paid or unpaid advertising, brochures, printed matter, directory listings, personal resumes or curriculum vitae, interviews or comments for use in media, statements in legal proceedings, lectures and public presentations, social media, and published materials.

RESEARCH

Any data-based activity designed to generate generalizable knowledge for the discipline, often through professional presentations or publications. The use of an experimental design does not by itself constitute research. Professional presentation or publication of already collected data are exempt from elements in section 9.0 (Behavior Analysts and Research) that pertain to prospective research activities (e.g., 9.02a). However, all remaining relevant elements from section 9.0 apply (e.g., 9.01 Conforming with Laws and Regulations; 9.03 Informed Consent Relating to Use of Client Data).

RESEARCH REVIEW BOARD

A group of professionals whose stated purpose is to review research proposals to ensure the ethical treatment of human research participants. This board might be an official entity of a government or university (e.g., Institutional Review Board, Human Research Committee), a standing committee within a service agency, or an independent organization created for this purpose.

RIGHTS AND PREROGATIVES OF CLIENTS

Rights and prerogatives of clients refers to human rights, legal rights, rights codified within behavior analysis, and organizational and administrative rules and regulations designed to benefit the client.

RISK-BENEFIT ANALYSIS

A risk-benefit analysis is a deliberate evaluation of the potential risks (e.g., limitations, side effects, costs) and benefits (e.g., treatment outcomes, efficiency, savings) associated with a given intervention. A risk-benefit analysis should conclude with a course of action associated with greater benefits than risks.

SERVICE RECORD

A client's service record includes, but is not limited to, written behavior-change plans, assessments, graphs, raw data, electronic recordings, progress summaries, and written reports.

STUDENT

A student is an individual who is matriculated at a college/university. This Code applies to the student during formal behavior-analytic instruction.

SUPERVISEE

A supervisee is any individual whose behavior-analytic services are overseen by a behavior analyst within the context of a defined, agreed-upon relationship.

SUPERVISOR

A supervisor is any behavior analyst who oversees behavior-analytic services performed by a supervisee within the context of a defined, agreed-upon relationship.

Appendix D: Considerations and Conversation Starters for RBT Trainers

The following scripts represent situations that RBTs may find themselves in from time to time; they are intended as exercises for in-service training sessions where there may be improv-like drills or role-plays to help RBTs bring up difficult conversations with their supervisors or handle situations with parents, strangers, administrators, or other therapists.

Code Section	Code Topic	Considerations and Conversation Starters
1.01	Upholding and prompting values and core principles of behavior analysis	Talk to your supervisor • "Can you give me some ideas on how to explain the difference between reinforcement and bribery to a teacher?" • "How do I get across the concept of consistency to a parent? I know this is a core principle of behavior analysis."

(*Continued*)

(Continued)

Code Section	Code Topic	Considerations and Conversation Starters
1.02	Remaining familiar with code	Talk to your supervisor • "To help me meet the ethics requirement of 1.02, I was wondering if we could review a new code section in our monthly meetings?" • "I would love to learn more about identifying and dealing with ethical dilemmas. Can we add the RBT Ethics Code to our standing supervision agenda?"
1.03	Be truthful and honest	Talk to an RBT colleague • "We need to talk about speaking honestly to parents; I think you might be giving them false hope with some of your comments." • "I think I need more honest feedback. You always say I'm doing fine, but I feel I've got a lot to learn."
1.04	Obey the law; follow ethical codes	Talk to the company owner • "A couple of the RBTs are vaping marijuana before they work with clients. Is there something you can do? I really don't want to work around this situation."
1.05	Bring conflicts to supervisor attention	Talk to your supervisor • "I have a problem with our policy of billing for the whole session when it is cut short. Can we talk?" • "I know our policy is 'Be nice to the clients,' but I believe Mr. Stuart is getting the wrong idea and is now texting me private messages."
1.06	Avoid multiple relationships	Talk to your supervisor's boss • "My supervisor is inviting her RBTs over for football night and other socials. This seems like a dual relationship to me, and now they are getting favors from her." • "The Fisher family is very friendly, and they want me to spend the weekend with them and their child at the beach. How do I handle this?"
1.07	No sexual relationships with clients or supervisors	Talk to your supervisor's supervisor • "My BCBA supervisor is coming on to me. It's very sexual and uncomfortable. I don't want to be rude, but if I refuse, I'm afraid he'll take me off the schedule or get me fired."

Code Section	Code Topic	Considerations and Conversation Starters
1.08	Personal problems and conflicts with others	Talk with your supervisor • "I've got a problem with Jamiya. Her cubicle is next to mine and she talks on the phone with her boyfriend all day. It's very distracting. Also, I think she is copying my behavior plans and using them with her clients." • "I think I'm having early signs of burnout. I feel tired and can't sleep, and at my last visit, my doctor said I had high blood pressure. Can you help me?"
1.09	Follow through on obligations	Talk with clinical director • "I've had an offer from a company across town that will pay me $2/hr more than what I am making here. I know I agreed to be with ABC Agency for at least one year, but this may be too good to pass up." • "I want to talk about switching clients. I'm not getting any results with my ASD clients; can I switch to the DD side?"
1.10	Do not make false public statements about work	Talk to an RBT colleague • "I saw your post on Facebook about your therapy with some of our clients. I believe in ABA, too, but to say that 'some are hopeless and some can be cured' doesn't seem right to me."
1.11	Provide current credentials to employers on request	Talk to your supervisor • "What credentials do you need to see for me to get promoted to Lead RBT? I've been here for 6 months now, and I believe I have had more success than anyone in our unit." • "I took the BCaBA exam on Friday, and I think I passed. Do I need to send you an email or something to get a pay increase?"
1.12	Obtain permission to use trademarks or copyrights	Talk to the BACB • "I would like to get permission to use some Board documents in a panel discussion at CalABA. How do I do that?"Talk to your supervisor • "Before I copy these assessments, I need to make sure I'm not going to get into trouble with the publisher. I see that there is a © symbol next to the words 'All Rights Reserved' at the bottom of each page."

(*Continued*)

(Continued)

Code Section	Code Topic	Considerations and Conversation Starters
1.13	Resolve issues informally; document efforts	Email to the ABAEthicsHotline • "How do I report my supervisor? I think she is violating Codes 5.04 and 5.06 of the Compliance Code. Her 'training' consists of handing out articles to read, and we never get any feedback. I haven't even seen her in the last month."
2.01	Support the legal rights and preferences of clients	Talk with parents • "I've been trying the reinforcers you suggested with Deon, but they don't seem to be working. I need to run a reinforcer assessment for the next couple of sessions to see what is going to work for him." Talk with supervisor. • "Ms. Catchum has been withholding Buster's lunch for no good reason that I can tell. What do I say to her? You know she's best friends with the principal, who is not going to do anything about this."
2.02	If those rights are violated, take necessary action	Phone call to child protective services • "Hello, my name is Lindsey, and I want to report a possible abuse of a client I work with. What information do you need?"Call to 911 • "Hello, we have a dangerous situation here; my client's father came home drunk, and he's waving a gun around,"
2.03	Do not discriminate against clients or other individuals or groups	Talk to supervisor • "I don't feel that I can give Layla the treatment she needs at the Ayub household. They are of a different religion and don't follow my beliefs at all. I love Layla to death and we really get along, but the parents are so critical of me and accuse me of all kinds of horrible things."
2.04	Do not accept gifts or give gifts to clients (or supervisors either)	Talk to parents • "I really appreciate your gift; this is so kind of you, but you know I can't accept this, and I hope you will understand." • "Look what Loren's family gave me for Valentine's Day. They are such sweet people. I'm willing to share the chocolates with the other RBTs on the team so it won't look like a gift just for me." • "I know you moved into a new home just recently, and I wanted you to have this bottle of wine from the Finger Lakes region where I went on vacation. It's Glenora Brut NV."

Code Section	Code Topic	Considerations and Conversation Starters
2.05	Do not share information about clients on social media	Talk to company owner • "One of the parents just told me that they are going to be featured on our company Facebook page along with their three kids. Did you know that this is a violation of our code of ethics?" • "I saw your photo on Facebook with your client Bruce. What gives? You know that is against the code, right?"
2.06	Always get permission to record interviews or client sessions	Talk to your supervisor • "Okay, so here is a short clip of me and Daniel, and as you can see, he is struggling with the 'mmm' sound." Supervisor: "Did you get permission to record this video? In writing?"
2.07	Protect confidential information about clients in your emails and reports	Talk to Lead RBT • "Hey, could you take a look at this report? It's my first one, and I wasn't sure of the format. I referred to the parents by their first names; I hope that is okay. Then I wasn't sure about the live-in mother-in-law; she babysits sometimes. How do I handle that?" (what is wrong with this?) • "I thought you would want to know; I just overheard a conversation between the parents, and I think they are going to separate. There was a lot of yelling, and Sgt. Spence was calling Laura all kinds of names. I think he might have PTSD."
2.08	Client information is on a need-to-know basis and only for job-related purposes	Talk with stranger at the park • "Yes, I am an autism specialist; how did you know? Oh, wait, I've got my company shirt on. I see. To answer your question, I'm working on manding with Wyatt today. He needs to learn to ask for things and not just point. This was his mother's idea . . . maybe you know her, Sam Harris—actually it's Samantha, but she said to just call her Sam."
2.09	Never disclose confidential information without consent of the client	Continued conversation with stranger at the park • "So anyway, where was I . . . oh yes, they might be moving from this neighborhood; they are really not happy with some of the people moving in."

(*Continued*)

(Continued)

Code Section	Code Topic	Considerations and Conversation Starters
2.10	Create, store, and dispose of records in a responsible manner	Talk with supervisor • "So, what do we do with all these paper records for Brenda now that her family is moving to Wyoming?" • My Lead RBT said I should scan these data sheets and then just toss the originals. Is that right? I thought I heard something about HIPAA-compliant procedures, whatever that is."
3.01	Practice only under close supervision of a qualified supervisor	Conversation with RBT colleague • "I'm not so sure about my supervisor; she doesn't ever give us a demonstration of what she wants us to do in our session. It's always, 'Well, this is a good time for you to start figuring some things out for yourself.' This doesn't give me confidence; is there any chance that she's really not qualified to supervise us? I heard it took her two times to pass the Board exam." • "I wanted you to know that I am so glad that I switched to you. My last supervisor was never around, and she made me fake the observations to make it look like I was getting my 5%."
3.02	Follow directions given by your supervisor; tell the supervisor if what he or she is asking goes beyond your Task List or competence	Talk to supervisor • "But I've never been involved in parent training before. I've only just worked in a clinic one-on-one with clients. I don't even know where to start working in-home teaching parents about behaviorism and contingencies of reinforcement."
3.03	RBTs must be competent in the methods and procedures that they provide for services	Talk to supervisor • "Yes, I've had experience with feeding programs. I actually spent the summer at the Penn State Children's Hospital Feeding Program in Hershey, and I would love to work on an in-home feeding program with Nick. Will you be my supervisor?"

Code Section	Code Topic	Considerations and Conversation Starters
3.04	Do not practice with new client populations unless you have training and supervision	Talk to parents • "You are very perceptive; I'm not very good with kids and don't know why they put me on this case. We are short-handed at the agency right now; maybe that's it." Talk to supervisor • "Is there any way that you can transfer me to another team? I'm not getting anywhere with the twins, the parents have noticed that I'm uncomfortable, and as I mentioned in my interview, I would rather work with adolescents."
3.05	Work only within the bounds of a written contract	Talk with your parents • "No, mom, I can't give you advice on how to deal with your nosy neighbor. I'm not allowed to; it's against my code of ethics." Talk with priest • "I'm so sorry, Father Murphy, I know those kids are noisy and rowdy during mass, but it's really up to the parents to control them. It sounds like a good idea that I would offer them some parent training since I'm a behavior specialist and all, but my code just won't allow that."
3.06	Talk to clients in plain English	Talk to supervisor • "So, you're saying that the parents reported me because they don't know what I'm talking about? What did they say? That I didn't explain Skinner's Three-Term Contingency properly? I started with a distinction between micro and macro contingencies. What can be more basic than that?"
3.07	Collect data accurately and display it so that it can be used in client program decision-making	Talk to BCaBA • "Okay, so I have all this frequency data. What's next? BCaBA: "Well, for starters, you should have been collecting interval data. There is no way to graph what we have here since you did not write down the start and stop times of your observations, and I seriously doubt that these high frequencies will produce acceptable IOA numbers." Talk to supervisor • "Where can I find something that will show me the proper graphing protocol for this data? The BCaBA seems to think that my data is no good, but I know I've seen frequency used in graphs before."

(*Continued*)

(Continued)

Code Section	Code Topic	Considerations and Conversation Starters
3.08	You should not be using non-behavior-analytic procedures. If you do, make sure that you do not imply you are doing it in the context of your work as an RBT.	Conversation with therapist • "So, you think that using this gravity blanket will somehow reduce my client's anxiety and depression as well? You know that I'm not allowed to work it into my ABA programming, right? Why? Well, it's not a behavior-analytic procedure." Phone conversation with parents • "Yes, I am able to babysit for you since you are not one of my clients, but you understand that I am not allowed to use behavioral procedures while I'm there with your son. I can play games, watch TV, and read to him, but I'm not allowed to set up or implement behavior programs. Okay, then; it was nice talking to you."

Bibliography

ABA Ethics Hotline (J. Bailey, Ed.). ABA Ethics Hotline.com. Retrieved December 29, 2019.

ABA Therapy Billing and Insurance Services (M. Silcox, Ed.). ABABilling.net. Retrieved December 29, 2019.

Agency for Persons with Disabilities (2008). The bill of rights for persons who are developmentally disabled. *State of Florida.* http://apd.myflorida.com/training/docs/bill-of-rights-2008.pdf. Retrieved December 29, 2019.

Americans with Disabilities Act of 1990, Pub. L. No. 101–336, 104 Stat. 328 (1990).

Atlantic Magazine (2018). What gifting rituals from around the globe reveal about human nature. www.theatlantic.com/sponsored/hennessy-2018/what-gifting-rituals-around-globe-reveal-about-human-nature/2044/. Retrieved December 29, 2019.

Autism Science Foundation (2019). *Beware of Non-Evidence-Based Treatments.* https://autismsciencefoundation.org/what-is-autism/beware-of-non-evidence-based-treatments/. Retrieved December 29, 2019.

BACB Newsletter (2017, April). *Appropriate RBT Activities.* www.bacb.com/wp-content/uploads/170421-newsletter.pdf. Retrieved December 29, 2019.

Baer, D. M., Wolf, M. M., & Risley, T. R. (1968). Some current dimensions of applied behavior analysis. *Journal of Applied Behavior Analysis, 1*, 91–97.

Bailey, J. S., & Burch, M. R. (2005). *Ethics for Behavior Analysts* (1st ed.). New York: Routledge.

Bailey, J. S., & Burch, M. R. (2011). *Ethics for Behavior Analysts* (2nd ed.). New York: Routledge.

Bailey, J. S., & Burch, M. R. (2016). *Ethics for Behavior Analysts* (3rd ed.). New York: Routledge.

Behavior Analyst Certification Board (2011). *Guidelines for Responsible Conduct*. Littleton, CO: Author.

Behavior Analyst Certification Board (2016). *Professional and Ethical Compliance Code for Behavior Analysts*. www.bacb.com/wp-content/uploads/BACB-Compliance-Code-english_190318.pdf. Retrieved December 29, 2019.

Behavior Analyst Certification Board (2018). *RBT Audit Documentation and Sample Supervision Log*. www.bacb.com/wp-content/uploads/RBT-Audit-Documentation-and-Supervision-Log-181227.pdf. Retrieved December 29, 2019.

Behavior Analyst Certification Board (2019a). *RBT Ethics Code*. www.bacb.com/wp-content/uploads/RBT-Ethics-Code_190227.pdf. Retrieved December 29, 2019.

Behavior Analyst Certification Board (2019b). *RBT Renewal Competency Assessment Packet: Requirements*. www.bacb.com/wpcontent/uploads/RBT_Competency_Assessment_Renewal_191030.pdf. Retrieved December 29, 2019.

Behavior Analyst Certification Board (2019c). *RBT Supervision and Supervisor Requirements*. www.bacb.com/wp-content/uploads/RBT-Supervision-and-Supervisor-Requirements_190529.pdf. Retrieved December 29, 2019.

Behavior Analyst Certification Board (2019d). *RBT Task List* (2nd ed.). www.bacb.com/wp-content/uploads/RBT-2nd-Edition-Task-List_181214.pdf. Retrieved December 29, 2019.

Behavior Analyst Certification Board (2019e). *Registry of Certificants*. www.bacb.com/find-a-certificant/. Retrieved December 29, 2019.

Behavior Analyst Certification Board (2019f). *Supervisor Training Curriculum Outline (2.0)*. www.bacb.com/wpcontent/uploads/Supervision_Training_Curriculum_190813.pdf. Retrieved December 29, 2019.

Equal Employment Opportunity Commission (1964). *Title VII of the Civil Rights Act of 1964*. www.eeoc.gov/laws/statutes/titlevii.cfm. Retrieved December 29, 2019.

Fabian-Weber, N. (2019). *8 Dangers of Social Media to Discuss with Kids and Teens*. www.care.com/c/stories/4275/5-dangers-of-social-media-to-discuss-with-you/. Retrieved December 29, 2019.

Florida Statutes. Florida patient's bill of rights and responsibilities. *Title XXIX*. Chapter 381. www.leg.state.fl.us/Statutes/index.cfm?App_mode=Display_Statute&URL=0300-0399/0381/Sections/0381.026.html. Retrieved December 29, 2019.

Jellies Blog. *5 Reasons Not to Post about Your Child on Social Media*. https://jelliesapp.com/blog/5-reasons-not-to-post-about-your-child-on-social-media. Retrieved December 29, 2019.

Journal of Applied Behavior Analysis. Wiley Online Library. https://onlinelibrary.wiley.com. Retrieved December 29, 2019.

Koocher, G. P., & Keith-Spiegel, P. (2008). *Ethics in Psychology and the Mental Health Professions: Standards and Cases* (3rd ed.). New York: Oxford University Press.

Legal Services Commission of South Australia. *Confidentiality: Duty to Maintain Confidentiality*. https://lawhandbook.sa.gov.au/ch29s03.php. Retrieved December 29, 2019.

Mauss, M. (2000). *The Gift: The Form and Reason for Exchange in Archaic Societies*. New York: WW Norton Co.

Mitchell, P. (2017). What predators look for when you post photos of your children online. *Parenting Magazine*. www.kidspot.com.au/parenting/teenager/cybersafety/what-predators-look-for-when-you-post-photos-of-your-children-online/news-story/9fea05351fdb8ab8c6bdea6acd8bfe60. Retrieved December 29, 2019.

National Library of Medicine. (2002). *Greek Medicine: The Hippocratic Oath* (M. North, Trans.). www.nlm.nih.gov/hmd/greek/greek_oath.html. Retrieved December 29, 2019.

Plunkett, L. A. (2019). *Sharenthood: Why We Should Think before We Talk about Our Kids Online*. Boston: MIT Press.

Schmitz, S., & Silcox, M. (2019). *Revenue Cycle Management ABA Therapy*. Buzzards Bay, MA: Cape Cod Collaboration.

Thyer, B. A. (2019). Pseudoscientific therapies for Autism Spectrum Disorder. In J. L. Matson (Ed.), *Handbook of Intellectual Disabilities, Autism and Child Psychopathology*. New York: Springer Nature Switzerland.

U.S. Department of Education (2015). *IDEA: Individuals with Disabilities Education Act*. https://sites.ed.gov/idea/#. Retrieved December 29, 2019.

Van Houten, R., Axelrod, S., Bailey, J. S., Favell, J. E., Foxx, R. M., Iwata, B. A., & Lovaas, O. I. (1988). The right to effective behavioral treatment. *Journal of Applied Behavior Analysis*, *21*(4), 381–384.

VB-MAPP. Verbal Behavior Milestones Assessment and Placement Program. *Mark Sundberg*. www.vbmappapp.com. Retrieved December 29, 2019.

Wallace, M., & Mayer, G. R. (2019). *Principles of Applied Behavior Analysis for Behavior Technicians (BTs) and Other Practitioners.* Cornwall on Hudson: Sloan Publishing.

Wikipedia.org. *Privacy Law.* https://en.wikipedia.org/wiki/Privacy_law. Retrieved December 29, 2019.

Index